Coping with

SKIN AND HAIR PROBI

Dr Judy Bury, the General Editor of this series, has worked in general practice and family planning for many years. She writes regularly on medical topics, and has a particular interest in self-help approaches to health care.

Other titles in the series include:

Coping with Caesarean and Other Difficult Births
Coping with Aging Parents
Coping with a Dying Relative
Coping with Sexual Relationships
Coping with Periods
Coping with Your Handicapped Child

Coping with
SKIN AND HAIR PROBLEMS

IRENE LEIGH,
BSc MB MRCP

FENELLA WOJNAROWSKA,
MA BSc BM BCh MRCP

With a Foreword by
Dr MICHAEL SMITH

Chambers

Published by W & R Chambers Ltd Edinburgh

Illustrations by A. Barrett

ISBN 0 550 20506 3

British Library Cataloguing in Publication Data

Leigh Irene
Coping with skin and hair problems.
1. Skin — Diseases 2. Hair — Diseases
3. Scalp — Diseases
I. Title II. Wojnarowska, Fenella T.
616.5 RL71
ISBN 0-550-20506-3

Printed by Clark Constable, Edinburgh, London, Melbourne

Contents

Dr Leigh is a consultant dermatologist at a London teaching hospital and has been specialising in dermatology for over twelve years. Her research interests are particularly laboratory based and concern psoriasis.

Dr Wojnarowska is a consultant dermatologist currently involved in both clinical dermatology and in clinical and experimental dermatology research. Her special interests are in acne and related problems.

Foreword

The skin and its appendages, the hair, nails and secretory glands or pores, constitutes the largest 'organ' of the body, although it is rarely thought of as such. It performs a wide range of functions. For example, it protects our body most effectively from the extremes of heat and dehydration, contamination from potentially poisonous dirt, and also the millions of sometimes harmful germs that we come into contact with every day. The skin exerts a fine control—it lets out just enough water in the form of perspiration to cool us down, but not so much that our body becomes dried out and unable to function. Abnormalities of the skin, since they are more noticeable than those of internal organs, can have an emotional and psychological effect upon us that can be out of all proportion to the size and degree of the disfigurement suffered. In short, our skin is vitally important to us whichever way you look at it!

Now, while a little learning has been said to be a dangerous thing, a little knowledge is always better than no knowledge. A lot of knowledge is better still and this book on skin and hair certainly contains that and presents it in both a concise and readable way. It should help you, reader, to understand better how most of the common skin problems arise, and should you have a skin problem yourself, the book should help you to understand better your doctor's explanation and treatment when you seek his advice.

Michael Smith
London, 1985

Introduction

The skin is a vital part of the body—it is an organ that most people take for granted until something goes wrong. Then we realise how important skin is for our self-image. People with skin disease make up a large percentage of the population. A 'leper' mentality still exists with regard to skin disease and unwittingly hurtful comments may be made which increase the suffering of those with skin problems and make them shun any activity requiring bare skin. Many skin diseases cause itching and discomfort for long periods of time. Severe skin disease may occasionally cause failure of the functions of the skin and this can be as serious as liver or kidney failure. We have included some of the most common skin diseases in this book in addition to information about the way sunshine, heat, cold and cosmetics affect the skin. However, to understand what happens when the skin *goes wrong* it is important to know how normal skin behaves so we start with some basic facts on skin.

1. Some Basic Facts

Functions of the skin

Protection

The outermost layer of the epidermis is a very hard horny layer which protects the more delicate tissues from injury. This hard layer is waterproof and forms a barrier to germs from the outside world. It is constantly being replenished by growth from the bottom growing layer of the epidermis which pushes cells upwards to the surface. Small fine scales are continuously shed from the surface and are not usually noticeable unless there is something wrong with the skin. The time taken for a skin cell to move from the growing layer to the outside is 14-21 days but this may be altered in skin diseases.

Response to Injury

Cuts and grazes to the skin are rapidly sealed by filling in the surface of the graze with clotted blood and then the growing layer starts to extend from the edges of the wound to bridge the gap. Without this efficient system, we would soon be invaded by outside germs.

Sweating

The specialised sweat glands of the body have several functions. The small glands secrete sweat to cool us down and to control the amount of fluid in the body. Some waste materials (from onions and garlic, for example) may be partly removed in the sweat. The larger sweat glands of the armpits and groin are under the control of our emotions. These give us our distinctive smell which with pheromones (specialised scents) play some part in physical attraction.

Lubrication

The grease glands of the body secrete an oil (sebum) which coats the skin, helping to protect it and kill germs. Androgens (male hormones) stimulate the glands to produce oil and they develop after puberty, when both men and women have more androgens in their blood. The amount of grease produced varies and some of us have oily skin and others may have dry skin because of variations in the response of the glands to androgen level.

Sensation

Nerves in the skin allow us to appreciate many different sensations: heat, cold, touch, pain, itching, pleasurable stroking, position and vibration. Loss of sensation due to nerve disease will lead to damage of the skin, e.g. if we were without sensations of pain and temperature, picking up a pan would lead to burning.

Sexual attraction and appearance

Idealisation of 'a flawless skin', emphasised in millions of adverts, romantic novels and newspapers, promotes the idea that this is important for sexual attractiveness and general appearance. People who feel their skin is flawed may withdraw from sexual relationships and from work which involves meeting the public.

Skin Colour

a) Colour cells (melanocytes) are studded in their millions throughout the skin. They produce a brown pigment called melanin which travels through elongated (dendritic) outgrowths of the cell wall into the surrounding skin cells of the growing (basal) layers where it protects them from the harmful effects of sunshine. All races have the same number of colour cells in the skin but they produce different amounts of pigment. In all races the colour production will be increased by sunshine.

b) Blood Supply. The colour of the skin also depends on the blood supply to the skin. An extensive network of blood vessels runs underneath the epidermis. These react to heat and cold (see Page 15). The blood vessels can open up as a result

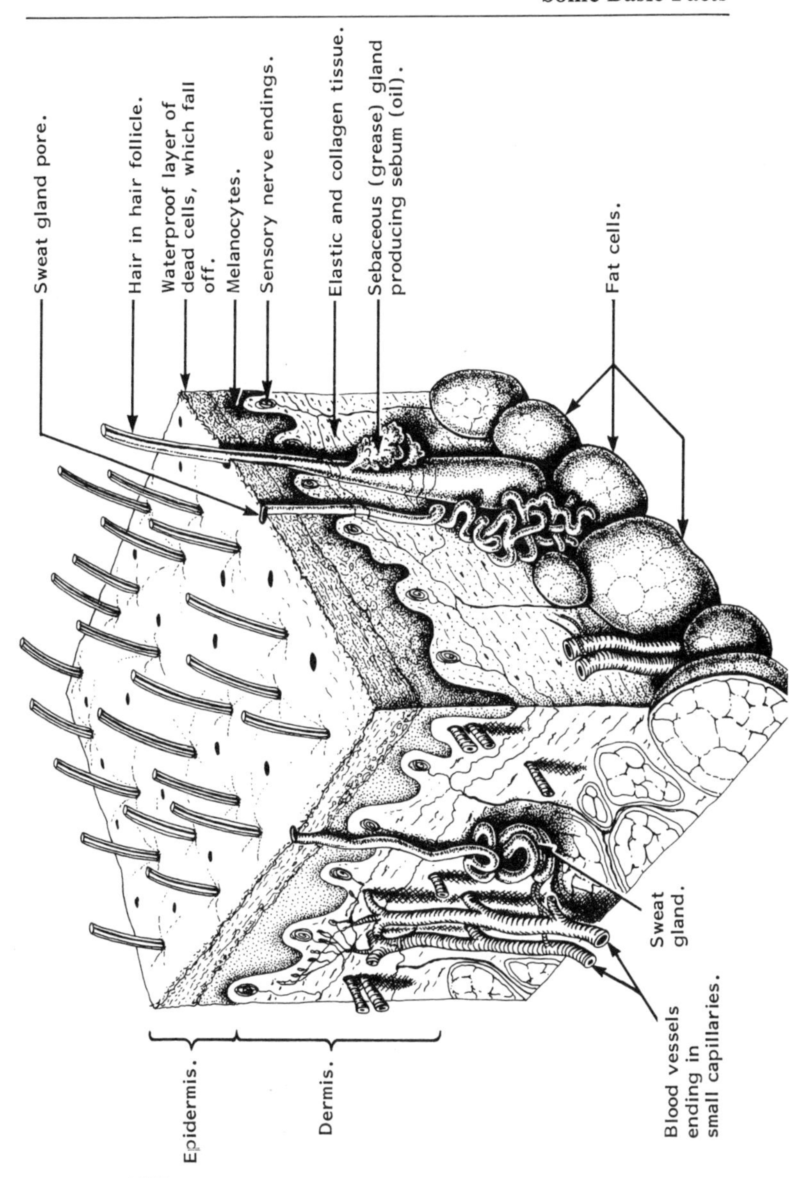

Diagram of Skin

The skin has several layers made up of different types of cells. The outer layers, the *epidermis*, have an underlying support network of elastic and strong collagen tissue called the *dermis*.

of emotion or embarrassment giving a 'blush', and hormone changes of the menopause can cause hot flushes.

A lot of blushing or sunshine may give permanently swollen blood vessels seen on the cheeks as reddish broken lines. This may be very marked in outdoor workers, giving a 'weathered appearance' with a continual high colour.

The Four Ages of the Skin

Throughout life the skin changes according to our age, mood, hormones and exposure to foods and chemicals. Therefore, at certain times we are prone to develop certain skin problems.

Infancy

In babies and infants skin bacteria can break down urine to produce ammonia which is very irritating to the skin and may cause a nappy rash. This forms sores and ulcers on the visible areas of skin (and not in the skin creases). It is very important always to wash the skin at each nappy change to remove the bacteria.

Many babies are prone to getting a rash which often looks like a bad nappy rash but also affects the creases of the bottom and is very red and crusted all over the bottom. This can also affect the creases of the body not covered by nappies—around the neck and under the arms, and these babies often have severe cradle cap. This is a form of eczema, known as seborrhoeic eczema of infancy. It will need the usual protective creams for babies' bottoms—zinc and castor oil, drapolene, etc., but it is also useful to avoid baby detergents and soaps and to use the detergent-free emulsifying ointment or aqueous cream (available from chemists) for washing.

Sometimes the rash becomes infected with thrush and small pustules are visible. Use of nystatin-hydrocortisone cream from the GP each time the nappy is changed soon cures this.

This form of eczema is not related to infantile eczema and usually disappears completely within a few months.

Babies who are kept too warm and become damp from sweating and urine often develop crops of red spots which may blister. These happen in skin folds and under nappies and are called prickly heat or sweat rash. The baby is uncomfortable. This will stop if the baby is kept cooler, especially if left without nappies for a few hours a day.

There is no medical condition known as 'teething rash'. Any rash that occurs during the early teething period (5-12 months) may be called this by mothers. Commonly, such rashes are due to virus infections which produce dramatic, alarming red rashes that quickly subside and have no lasting ill-effects. Strong antiseptic creams—Germolene, Savlon, Dettol—should be avoided as they will make the rash worse.

Milk spots may be a cause of alarm to a new mum or dad, especially with first babies. They are tiny spots which appear on both cheeks. They are normal between the ages of 2-6 weeks and are due only to the immaturity of the skin glands and hormone changes. It is best to leave them alone as cream and greases will make them last longer and they will soon disappear on their own.

Infancy is also the age when atopic eczema starts (see Chapter 2).

Adolescence

The major affliction of adolescence is the tendency to develop acne, which affects every teenager once puberty has started. As this is so visible, teenagers may be very upset about their appearance and very uncooperative about treatment. It is important to take acne seriously and to treat it quickly to prevent scarring (see Chapter 3).

Another problem may be the enlargement of birthmarks or an increased awareness of birthmarks, at a time of developing relationships with the opposite sex. They may become an obsession, even if they are barely noticeable to the outside observer. Many birthmarks look better than the results of trying to remove them. In any case all surgery should be left until adult years to lessen scarring.

Male pattern baldness may develop in late teenage years and is a further affront to young male vanity. Little can be done to ease this.

Rapid growth in height or weight may give rise to stretch marks on the trunk and limbs. These will be worsened by additional physical stress, e.g. weightbearing. There is little that can be done to slow down growth in height, but a suitable diet for those tending to overweight will help.

Adulthood

Stretch marks appear in skin when there is a rapid increase in weight. They are cracks in the supporting network of the skin, and they remain when the weight is lost so it is best to avoid them. Pregnancy is obviously associated with a drastic weight change and so stretch marks appear on the tummy. Creams will not affect the development of stretch marks, nor does surgery help, so try to avoid putting on too much weight—don't eat for two! Thin women have less room for expansion so are more affected than fat women.

Pregnancy is also a time when the hair changes—less hair falls out so the hair is thicker than usual. High levels of hormones inhibit acne spots and cause swollen blood vessels to become apparent as red marks, and may cause swelling of the hands and feet. Unfortunately, these hormones also stimulate colour production of the skin. In addition to darkening of the nipple, umbilicus and lines on the tummy, dark brown patches may appear on the face (melasma). These will improve after the pregnancy but can be helped by avoiding sunshine on the face. Itching is often a problem in pregnancy and usually occurs without a rash, but may keep women awake as itching is always worse when the skin warms up at night. Other skin rashes change in pregnancy —psoriasis often gets better but eczema may get worse because of the itching.

'Housewives' hands' are a hazard to the mother (and father) after the baby is born. Exposure to too much soap powder and detergents gives a dry cracking eczema of the hands (see Chapter 2).

Aging

As we age the skin becomes thinner both in the outer layer and in the supporting tissue so the skin wrinkles and becomes less elastic. This is increased by exposure to sun so is often noticeable initially on the neck and face. A yellowish mottling occurs with yellowish lumps with a scraggy appearance on the sides of the neck ('Berkshire' or 'chicken neck'). The blood vessels lose some support and so bruising happens very easily, even without injury to the skin. Bruises last a long time on the arms. The skin produces fewer protective oils and so is very prone to dry out with soap and detergents. Overbathing, especially with foam bath, may give a very dry and itchy skin. Older skin tends to develop lumps and bumps—warts, skin tags, freckles, white patches and skin cancers. Swollen blood vessels give tiny red spots. Most of these are harmless but lumps which continue to increase in size or colour should be checked by a doctor. Hair thinning may occur all over the scalp, but usually is worse over the front.

Sunshine and Your Skin

There have been reports in women's magazines and newspapers of the harmful effects of sunbathing. However, sunshine adds more to our enjoyment of our summer holidays and many of us travel far afield to be sure of the sunshine. What are we to think about these opposing viewpoints and how should they influence our behaviour? Is our summer holiday going to do us any harm? For most of us a sensible course depends on understanding ultraviolet radiation and our skin type.

What is Ultraviolet Radiation? (UVR)

We can neither see nor feel ultraviolet radiation from the sun—it is neither heat nor light.

Direct exposure to ultraviolet radiation can damage the eye (e.g. at the eclipse of the sun). The amount of ultraviolet depends on the distance from the equator and on the altitude. In Great Britain the UVR increases in summer and is maximal between 11 am and 3 pm regardless of weather conditions. Nearer the equator and higher up mountains, the amount of UVR and sun damage will be proportionately greater.

Tanning and skin types

UVR stimulates the colour cells (melanocytes) of the skin to produce a brown pigment (melanin) which absorbs UVR and protects the skin from damage by a suntan and by skin thickening. People vary in their ability to tan and this has led to a classification of skin types listed below.

Type I —never tan, always burn (often red hair— Celtic)
Type II —always burn, sometimes tan
Type III —sometimes burn, always tan
Type IV —never burn, always tan
Type V —pigmented skin

People with Skin Type I must always protect their skin from sunshine as they have a high risk of sun damage. However, as the skin type number increases the skin protects itself by tanning.

It is *never* necessary to burn to produce a suntan—indeed severe sunburn will blister and will result in the loss of skin and tan. Sunburn may also be one of the predisposing factors to malignant moles.

Beneficial effects of UVR

In many parts of the world a pale skin is desirable; in the West

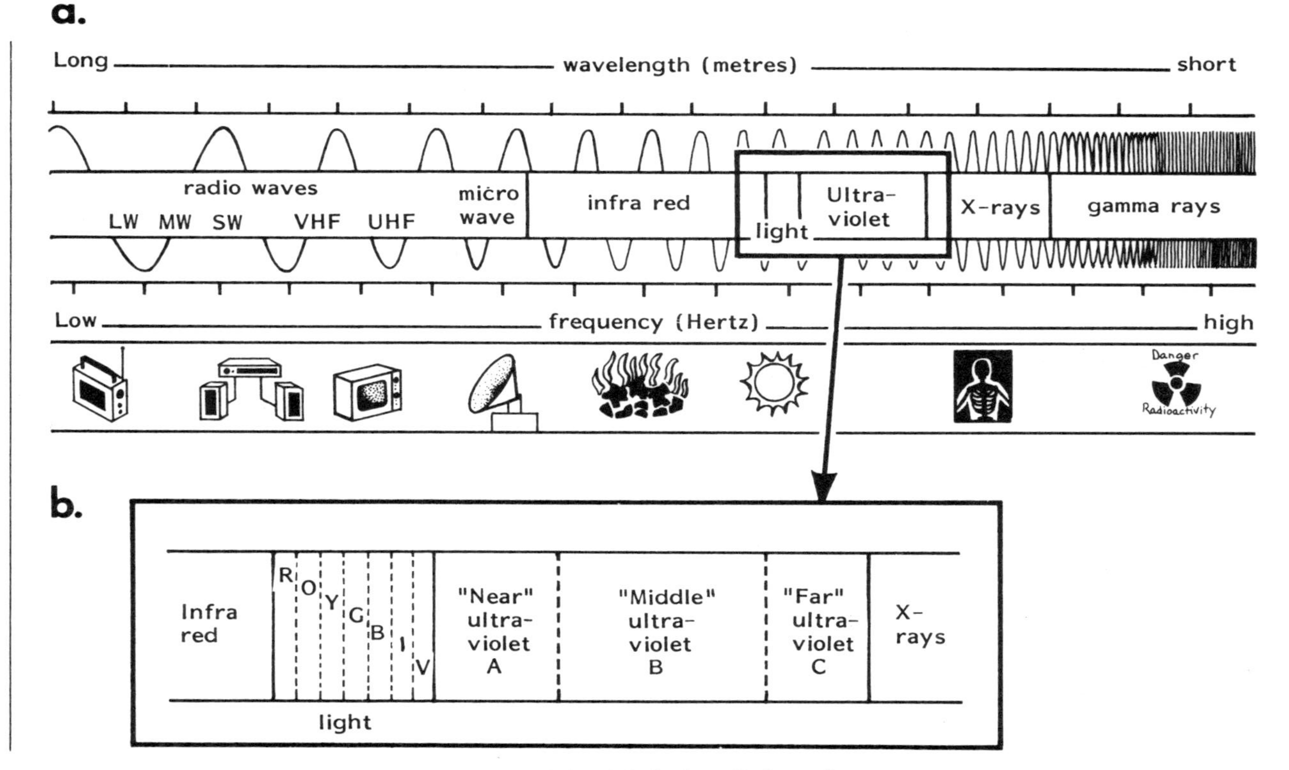

The position of ultraviolet in the radiation scale.

suntanned is beautiful. Sunbathing is pleasurable and makes us feel more attractive. A beneficial effect is that our skin can synthesise Vitamin D, preventing rickets.

Harmful Effects of U V R

Skin Cancer

The skin cell is continuously damaged by U V R and repairs itself. These mechanisms are very efficient but mistakes appear with age and abnormal cells eventually develop into skin cancers (see Chapter 5). Elderly people who have lived in the tropics, worked out of doors or have Type I skin are especially at risk.

Sun freckles

Harmless lumps and bumps also appear on sun-exposed skin. These include freckles, pale white patches and rough scaly keratoses. They are cosmetic problems only and can be removed easily but most people who get them, get lots of them.

Aging

U V R damages the elastic and supporting tissue of the skin, which loses its elasticity and tends to wrinkle, accentuating the changes of aging.

Allergies to U V R

Skin allergies to U V R tend to appear on the sun-exposed sites (see Diagram). The commonest allergy to U V R is called polymorphic light eruption and may affect 10% of the population, women more than men. U V R is the cause and the rash appears during the summer months. In many people the rash is mild and wrongly called heat bumps or prickly heat. It usually consists of juicy red spots, especially on the arms and hands, which appear in the evening after 1-2 hours of sun exposure and last 7-10 days. Repeated sunbathing lessens the reaction so the rash will tend to wear off as summer progresses. In many, the rash only appears with intense sunbathing but it can ruin holidays.

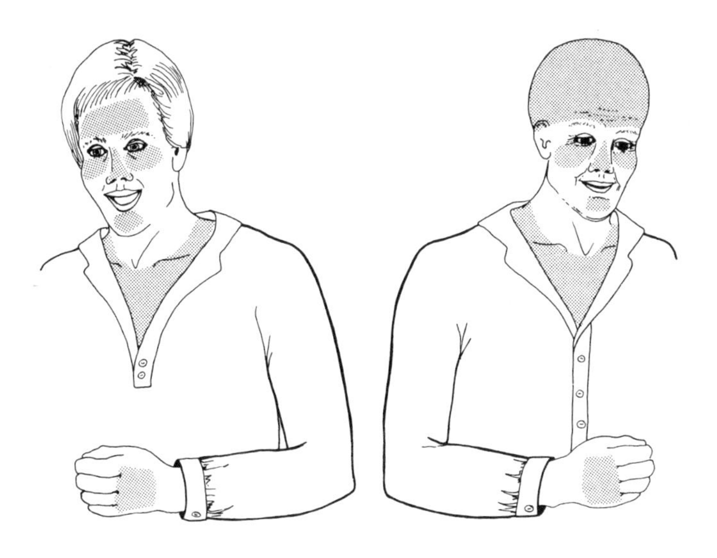

Sun-exposed sites.

There are many photosensitive allergies due to perfumes and drugs (see Chapter 2), and a few people develop eczema in sun-exposed sites (see Diagram) due to allergy to UVR. The clue to all these rashes lies in their distribution on the skin—if they are on the sun-exposed sites, suspect sunlight.

How to protect your skin

It is important to recognise your skin type. If you are fair-skinned, you should protect your skin with clothing and sun-blocking creams as much as possible and avoid direct sunshine. By all means sit on the beach but under an umbrella. If you have an allergy to sunshine then avoid being out of doors between 11 am and 3 pm as much as possible whatever the weather, because it's better to be outside on a sunny evening than a cloudy midday. Wear a hat with a brim and long-sleeved clothing.

There are many sunblocking creams which are very

effective. The strength is indicated by the sun protection factor SPF—the higher the SPF the longer you can be out of doors (see lists below).

Sunscreens

High Sun Protection Factor (SPF)

Spectraban forte
Piz Buin
  Extreme Cream No. 6/8
Coppertone
  Super Shade No. 15
Delial 10
ROC 10

Low SPF

Uvistat
Innoxa 12W
Ritz Bronze

Medium SPF

Lancome Hydra Bronze
ROC Sunscreen Creams
Skol Cream
Germaine Monteil Strong
Ambre Solaire Cream
Nivea Sunfilter Cream
Eversun Milk
Avon Bronze Cream

These creams should be applied at frequent intervals whilst out of doors. Even if you have Type III or IV skin, harmful effects can be reduced by using mild protection creams (low SPF) and gentle exposure without burning until a tan develops.

Tan promoters

Some suntan lotions contain plant products (e.g. bergamot) which increase tanning. They are used medically in PUVA (see Chapter 3). They probably increase the risk of skin cancer and skin aging. Vitamin tablets are useless in promoting tanning or preventing sunburn.

Fake suntans

Fake suntans result from a chemical (dihydroxyacetone) which stains the skin surface and will wear off with time. The colour is an orangey brown and can be streaky if not evenly applied. This chemical provides no protection against burning, so a sunblocking cream should be used in addition for sunbathing.

Sunbeds and UV Lamps

UV lamps used to be mainly of sunburn wavelengths (UVB) and tended to produce burning with over-exposure. New fluorescent tubes emit UVA which does not burn (although it can produce itching and flushing). They will not prevent burning with natural sunlight. These have been marketed as sunbeds and are popular in salons and beauty parlours. They cannot tan skin which normally will not tan. Sunbeds produce harmful UVR effects on the skin with time, in particular skin aging, freckling, and possibly skin cancer, and repeated or prolonged use should be avoided. It is essential *always* to protect the eyes, which can be damaged, when using any sunbed or UV lamp. Also wash off perfumes before usage.

Check that you are not taking any medicines which make you sensitive to sunlight.

Summary

Prolonged UVR can be harmful to the skin but limited exposure (summer holidays, for example) with avoidance of sunburn, gradual tanning and sensible protective measures will produce little harm unless you have an allergy to sunshine. However, it is important to recognise the limitations of your skin type.

Heat and Cold on your Skin

The skin reacts to heat and cold in many ways. Most reactions are to the body's advantage, but some are troublesome and a few are dangerous.

The body needs a constant internal temperature for all its processes to function properly. The skin regulates the body temperature by reducing loss of heat when the outside is cold or losing extra heat when the body is too hot. We assist the skin in doing this by altering our clothing.

Heat and Your Skin

Coping with heat

Hot weather, warm clothes or a fever cause the body temperature to rise, and set off the heat-losing mechanisms of the skin, which are:

Reddening of the skin due to enlarging of blood vessels. The blood is warm and loses heat to the surrounding air. The skin appears red and flushed, and feels warm to the touch.

Swelling of the skin. The enlarged blood vessels leak watery fluid which seeps into the skin (oedema) so rings and shoes become tight and ankles swell.

Sweating. The body cools itself by evaporating sweat from the skin. This is the most important way of losing heat. People who cannot sweat collapse from heat stroke in warm conditions.

Reactions to heat

Many people say they have suffered from 'heat rash'. There is no medical condition called 'heat rash', but there are several rashes that are caused by heat. Sun-induced rashes are often wrongly blamed on the heat rather than the sunlight.

Prickly heat (Miliaria)

When the body is hot, sweating occurs. In hot humid conditions and, in babies who are kept at tropical temperatures, under damp nappies, the sweat does not evaporate and swells the skin, causing blockage of the entrance to the sweat pores. This causes minute clear blisters, filled with sweat, which then burst and dry up.

If the sweat duct blocks deeper down, this is a serious condition. The sweat glands burst deep into the skin and are seen as small red bumps and blisters. They are very itchy and uncomfortable.

The only treatment that works is to keep cool in an air-conditioned room or a well-ventilated room.

The sweat ducts may remain blocked for weeks, and during

that time that area of skin cannot sweat. A person who has suffered widespread prickly heat cannot lose heat by sweating and develops 'heat stroke' or 'heat collapse'.

Heat and sweat allergy

A few unfortunate people break out in nettle rash (urticaria) as a reaction to raising the body temperature. In conditions that cause sweating, e.g. dancing, sports, hot baths and hot weather, tiny itchy bumps appear on the skin. Antihistamine tablets such as Phenergan or Piriton from the chemist, taken ½ hour before bathing, may help but will make you drowsy. Showers rather than hot baths may help.

Mottling from heat

Sitting too near open fires may cause a mesh of redness and discolouration on the legs which doesn't fade when away from the heat. This is a chronic low grade burn and it can also be produced on the tummy by hot water bottles.

Burns

Heating the skin causes a burn. Burns are classified as:

First Degree Burns. These mild superficial burns cause redness of the skin and later peeling. No treatment is necessary. Calamine lotion is soothing. They heal without scarring but there may be temporary darkening or lightening of the skin. Plunging the burnt area in cool water will not lessen the amount of damage but may numb the pain. Traditional remedies such as applying butter cannot reduce the burn and only make a mess!

Second Degree Burns. These are more severe, with blistering, swelling and redness of the skin. The blister may be burst with a needle (which has been sterilised in a flame) if uncomfortable. The burn should be kept clean and dry, and covered with sterile dressing if necessary. Creams are not necessary and can be harmful. There may be colour change for some months, but no permanent scarring.

Third and Fourth Degree Burns. These are very serious problems. The whole skin and underlying fat, muscle and tendons are burnt—sometimes down to the bone. The burn is black and charred, and painless, as the nerves are destroyed.

Such burns always require medical attention because of shock and later infection.

The complete destruction of the affected skin results in severe scarring when the burn heals.

Cold and your skin

Coping with cold

Cold activates the body's heat-saving mechanisms. In evolution we have lost the fur coat of our primate ancestors, so we compensate with warm clothing. The body core is kept warm at the expense of the skin, so that we develop frostbite before losing our vital functions.

Blue with cold

The skin loses heat from warm blood in the skin. When the body is cold the skin blood supply is cut down to reduce loss of heat. The blood is stagnant and becomes blue. This effect is most obvious in the fingers, toes, nose and ears. In plump women it appears on the thighs and upper arms as a blue mottled network because fat is a good insulator of the body, and the skin becomes colder first.

'Goose Pimples'

In our efforts to fluff out our non-existent fur coats we contract the muscles of the hair roots, forming 'goose pimples'. When the hairs stand on end they trap a layer of air between them which helps insulation.

Clothing for cold weather

Heat is lost chiefly from the face, hands, feet, and in babies and bald men from the head. Babies and bald men should wear bonnets or hats in cold weather. Gloves are very important for warmth and protection of the hands from chapping and chilblains (see next section). Warm socks or shoes are also essential. Layers of clothing, particularly of natural fibres such as cotton and wool, trap air which is a good insulator. Several layers of clothes are better than one thick garment because there will then be more layers of trapped air.

Reactions to cold

Chapping. Cold alters the structure of the horny outer layer of the epidermis making it dry and cracked. The skin may develop deep splits (fissures) which are very painful. Warm gloves and liberal use of hand creams both before and after cold exposure prevent this problem.

Winter Itch. In winter, the skin (especially on the legs) becomes dry and finely cracked with a crazy paving appearance. This is itchy and uncomfortable. It results from a combination of cold damage, drying out of the skin by the hot dry air of central heating and too much bathing.

The skin should be greased or moisturised regularly, and bathing reduced (see Chapter 5).

Chilblains. Chilblains affect the fingers and toes and, rarely, the thighs, particularly in horse riders and motor cyclists. The damaged areas become red, swollen, itchy and painful or burning. In severe cases they may blister and ulcerate. There is no treatment. Prevention is by wearing warm clothing and shoes to protect the area from the cold. Calcium and vitamins are useless. Smoking may make it worse. Once the skin has been damaged the speed of warming up the skin makes no difference, so prevention is the only way to deal with chilblains.

Dead Fingers (Raynaud's Phenomenon). The fingers and toes sometimes react to cold by going white, then blue and red on rewarming. The sensation is dulled whilst they are white and they may be very painful whilst warming up. Vibrating machinery such as drills, hair dryers and electric beaters can cause the same changes. Smoking makes this much worse. The only preventive measures are to wear warm gloves, socks and boots, to avoid vibration and to stop smoking.

Cold Urticaria. Cold is a very rare cause of nettle rash (urticaria). The skin reacts to cold by itching and forming weals. It is dangerous because sudden exposure to severe cold (for example the sea or swimming pool) may cause collapse.

Treatment from a specialist with drugs other than antihistamine tablets is often needed.

2. Eczema and Allergies

Atopic Eczema in Babies and Children

People who suffer from wheezing (asthma), hayfever, attacks of conjunctivitis (red, itchy eyes), or atopic eczema are called atopic. If unlucky, they may have more than one of these conditions. They may also suffer from urticaria in response to food or drugs, and usually have relatives with the same problems.

Allergy testing is often requested by eczema sufferers. Such tests give clues to factors triggering hayfever and asthma but eczema is a different type of reaction which is known as 'delayed hypersensitivity' as it occurs at 24-48 hours. Thus prick tests (see Chapter 3) are not relevant to eczema even though they may be positive. Trying to avoid substances which gave positive prick tests may help asthma or hayfever but not eczema. Allergy clinics may get carried away with prick test results.

Children very rarely have eczema due to contact allergy so the patch tests done for the 'delayed' reaction of contact eczema are not useful either.

Atopic eczema appears between 3 and 12 months of age and may persist into the teens, but most children get better earlier than this. The skin is very dry and the patches of eczema may be dry, red and scaly or weeping, and sometimes split. It is terribly itchy and the children are often disfigured by scratch marks. They also rub at the eczema, making the skin thick and ridged (lichenified).

The face, especially around the mouth and eyes, and the joints are particularly affected. In Asian and black children the rash is often very 'pebbly'. The skin in the areas of eczema may darken or lighten. There is no permanent colour change or scarring.

Coping with eczema

Treatment of eczema is aimed at making it less troublesome. Treatments cannot cure it but it will go away on its own, eventually.

Diet

Diets are fashionable. Breast-feeding only for the first 6-9 months has been recommended to prevent eczema. Many mothers have been needlessly made to feel guilty about bottle-feeding their baby, when this is still not proven to be harmful.

A few babies and children improve dramatically on a very strict diet free from cows' milk and eggs. There is no test of the blood or skin to show who will respond. Itching of the mouth on eating the food can be a pointer. The diet can lead to vitamin and calcium deficiency, and must only be done under medical supervision. It should be abandoned if there is no clear benefit in a two-month trial.

House dust mite

Most dust in bedding, curtains, carpets and soft furnishings contains large quantities of house dust mite (*dermatophagoides pteronyssines*). Allergy to this makes eczema worse in some people. Dust avoidance involves removal (this must not be done by the person concerned) of soft furnishings, curtains, carpets and ornaments; covering or replacing the mattress and using feather-free and washable bedding. Beds and room must be vacuumed daily and bedding washed once a week. Carpets must be removed from all areas where children lie or crawl.

Clothing

Wool, nylon and artificial fabrics make the skin more itchy and the eczema worse. Cotton clothes and sheets are very helpful.

Bathing

Soaps are drying to the skin but a *cool* bath with a special cleanser to grease the skin, like aqueous cream or emulsifying ointment, is very helpful. Oils may be added to the bath. Bubble baths are very drying and should be avoided.

Chlorinated swimming pools dry the skin and a shower after swimming to wash off the chlorine is essential. Sea bathing does not make eczema worse.

Heat and Weather

Heat makes eczema more itchy so baths and bedrooms should be cool and bedclothes should be kept to a minimum. Hot humid weather often makes eczema worse but sunlight is often beneficial. Cold winter weather and a hot, dry atmosphere due to central heating make the skin drier, cracked and more itchy.

Stress

It is common for eczema to flare when there's a family upset, when parents are not getting on, with jealousy of brothers and sisters, exams, change of school or any unhappiness or failure.

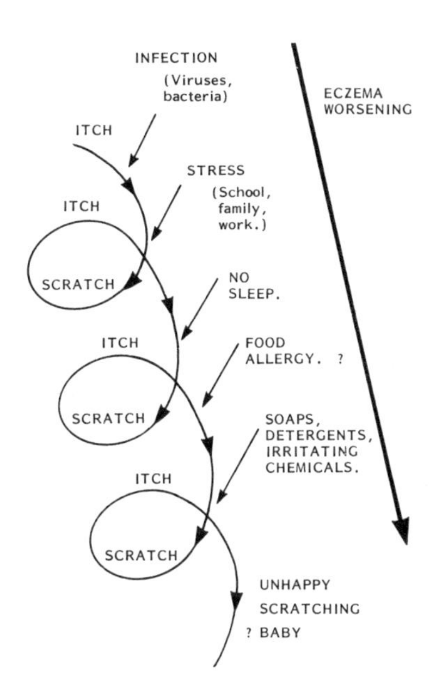

Stress and unhappiness both make eczema worse, but do not cause it. In addition bad eczema makes children miserable and irritable, and their parents get tense. As the eczema improves and everyone relaxes and can sleep at night, the children are transformed.

Holidays

The combination of relaxation, warmth and sunlight on holiday often transforms the child with eczema. The eczema may completely, though temporarily, clear.

Medicines

Doctors will prescribe steroid ointments which reduce the inflammation and itch in eczema, but only mild steroid ointments such as hydrocortisone can be used in babies. Hydrocortisone will be available without prescription shortly. In older children, stronger ointments can be used, although large amounts of steroids may thin the skin and, by passing through the skin, stop bone growth.

Coal tar or other medicated bandages used overnight are messy and unpleasant but they are very effective, especially for thick patches of chronic eczema.

Antihistamines taken at night reduce the itch and make the child drowsy, helping the child—and thus the whole family—to sleep.

Immunisations

All the normal childhood immunisations should be given *except* smallpox. Smallpox vaccination can be fatal in children with eczema.

Outlook

Eczema comes and goes for many years. Most children grow out of it, the eczema clearing between the ages of 2 and 10. It is impossible to predict when any particular child will be clear.

Optimism is essential. Parents and children get despondent, regarding eczema as a life sentence. Holidays, with their miraculous though short-lived effects, are important to restore morale to the whole family and convince them that the skin can and will return to normal. The relaxation of holidays is what benefits the child and moving home to the seaside will not do this.

A Useful Address:

The National Eczema Society provides help and advice on living with and managing eczema, including practicalities such as where to buy cotton clothing and goats' milk. They have a regular news-sheet and meetings with active local support groups. Contact:

National Eczema Society,
Tavistock House North,
Tavistock Square,
London WC1 9SR.

Eczema in Adults

Eczema is an intensely itchy rash, which varies from acute redness, swelling and blistering, with weeping crusted areas, to dry scaly patches, thick patches, and splits. There are many kinds of eczema. Atopic eczema is rare in adults but similar to the disease in children, contact allergic eczema is commoner. The other most important types are described below:

Hand and Foot Eczema

Eczema affecting the hands and feet is very disabling as it interferes with work, walking, hobbies and sports.

'Housewives' Hands'

Housewives, particularly those with babies and small children, often suffer dreadfully from very severe chapping of their hands. The hands get dry, red, cracked and sore.

Constant exposure to detergents, washing-up liquid, washing powder, bleaches, cleansing fluids and abrasives combined with continuous wetting, cold weather and the dry air of central heating degrease, damage and dry out the skin. Hairdressers doing repeated shampooing also suffer in this way.

The hands can be improved by protection and care, but it takes months for them to return to normal once damaged.

Contact with water must be avoided and rubber gloves used for all wet work and contact with detergents. Any soap, etc. must be very thoroughly rinsed off the hands and removed from beneath rings, then the hands carefully dried and greasy hand cream liberally applied. Cotton gloves protect during housework, and gloves should always be worn outside in cold weather.

Blistering Eczema of the Hands and Feet

Some unfortunate people have a very distressing blistering eczema of the palms or soles. The attacks start as tiny itchy blisters which dry to form peeling, itchy, cracked skin. The skin heals in one or two weeks. There may be a single attack or attacks may occur every few weeks for months or years. Frequent attacks may appear to be related to periods, but keeping a diary will show that this is not a constant relationship. It often disappears as suddenly as it started.

The cause is unknown, although stress, heat and sweating all may trigger attacks. Treatment helps the symptoms, but cannot prevent attacks. In the blistering stage soaking the hands or feet in cool potassium permanganate solution (diluted 1 in 8,000 to a pale pink colour) for 15 minutes and letting them dry in the air twice daily is soothing and prevents infection. A steroid ointment from your doctor can be applied both after the soaks and in the peeling stage as this reduces the itch and discomfort. The hands must be treated with care (see previous section). With treatment most people are able to live their normal lives.

Discoid Eczema

Many people have dry scaly itchy patches on their limbs or body. These may occasionally be severe and blister or weep, but are often only a minor discomfort. Their cause is unknown, but often stress makes them worse.

Steroid ointments prescribed by your doctor applied two to three times per day will suppress them. They tend to come and go for years before clearing.

Lichen Simplex

People with an atopic background may develop a thick patch of eczema in one place, usually the nape of the neck or leg. It is the result of an itch—scratch cycle; the skin itches, the person scratches, the skin thickens and itches more, and so on. It is an expression of stress and habit. Covering the patches may break the cycle, but often steroid ointments, tapes and/or injections into the patch to stop the itch are also required.

Seborrhoeic Eczema

This is the most common form of eczema. It is usually a minor nuisance but can be severe. Seborrhoeic eczema takes the form of dandruff with occasional redness and itching of the scalp, eyebrows and eyelashes. There may also be patches on the eyelids (often wrongly blamed on make-up), face, beard area and behind the ears, centre of the chest and back, and body folds, i.e. armpits, groins, under the breasts. It affects the pubic area (dandruff of the pubic hair), the genitals and the area around the back passage, causing redness, scaling, itching, discomfort and embarrassment. Dandruff is a noticeable increase in the normal shedding of fine scales from the scalp (see Chapter 4).

We do not know the cause of seborrhoeic eczema. Heat and sweating in skin folds make it worse but treatment is usually very successful, although it has to be continued for a long time. Dandruff can often be controlled simply by shampooing the hair every one to two days using coal tar, selenium sulphide or zinc pyrithione-containing shampoos (Polytar, Selsun, Head and Shoulders, Revlon Medicated). Sometimes an overnight treatment with sulphur and salicylic acid cream to the scalp is necessary. Creams should be applied to the scalp by parting the hair and rubbing the cream on the scalp which has been exposed, then reparting 1″ away and reapplying cream until the scalp has been covered. You may use hydrocortisone ointment on the face two to three times per day but this is the *only* steroid ointment which should be used. Stronger steroids such as Betnovate, Synalar, Dermovate and Propaderm will damage the delicate facial skin causing thin skin, damaged blood vessels and acne-like spots. Expensive cosmetic preparations often do not help and delay medical advice. When the eczema is present the face often cannot tolerate make-up, but as it subsides make-up can be worn without discomfort. Often patch testing (see page 30) is valuable to make sure that you are not allergic to make-up and cream and need not abandon them.

These different types of eczema should all be shown to your doctor who will help to differentiate them from allergic eczema and prescribe appropriate treatment. Many over-the-counter creams are useless and some will only make things worse by irritating the skin or causing allergic reactions. Simple soothing creams such as E45, oilatum cream and aqueous creams may help, as will bathing with emulsifying ointment, oilatum or Neutrogena soaps and oils. Hydrocortisone creams from the chemist may help mild cases. Avoid all antiseptics, either as creams or baths; stop bubble baths and bath salts as they will irritate the skin. Do not use Anthisan, Caladryl, Locan, Lanacaine or Boots antihistamine cream as these can cause allergies.

The Experience of Eczema

'There are four degrees of irritation: the slight itch everyone has now and then; a spasmodic itch which eventually goes; a hot itch which is initially relieved by scratching, but then increases; and an overwhelming hot flush that sends one up the wall. This fourth type, I found, leads to sleepless nights; you feel wet because the wounds are bleeding or weeping, and this means that you stick to the sheets. Scratching always seems worst at nights; sometimes you feel you want to rip the flesh from your bones.

Sleepless nights leave you unable to think straight; you are frustrated because you are always uncomfortable; and the lack of confidence because of your appearance completes the vicious circle of depression.

Some people find that special diets help; personally I have found them time-consuming and expensive, with little lasting effect. Antihistamines can help (though they don't after years of taking them); even when they do, once they wear off the irritation is doubled. It is a good idea to cut your nails short to minimise the damage you do while scratching.

I found I was able to control my scratching by keeping as clinically clean as possible. I make sure my skin is always moist; I put emulsion on my skin, and bath practically every night, with a water-dispersible oil as well as something to kill the bacteria in the water, and do not use soap or a flannel.'

Steroid Creams and Ointments

Weak (safe on face and babies)

Hydrocortisone	will be available off prescription

Moderate

Eumovate
Ultralanum
Haelan

Strong

Betnovate	can be diluted
Propaderm	so that it is less strong
Synalar	

Very Strong

Dermovate
Nerisone Forte

Allergies and the Skin

Allergies are fashionable and many people assume their skin trouble is due to an allergy but this is rarely true. Under 5 per cent of all patients attending skin clinics are suffering from a true allergy.

An allergic rash can be caused by a substance coming into contact with the skin (contact allergy), or can be a reaction to something entering the body.

Allergy to substances in contact with the skin (Contact Allergy)

There are two kinds of contact allergy — eczema and nettle rash.

Contact Eczema (Contact Dermatitis)

This is the commonest type of allergy. The skin reacts to contact with a substance (the allergen) by becoming red and itchy. In a very severe reaction the skin blisters or weeps. Swelling may be marked and may close the eyes if the face is affected. The skin becomes dry and scaly in more chronic cases. All these reactions are typical of eczema. This type of eczema occurs at the site of contact with the allergen, especially in areas where the skin is thin, such as the eyelids and backs of hands. The thick palms and soles are rarely affected by contact allergic rashes. Contact allergy is more likely to occur if the skin is broken or damp.

Contact allergy may develop to something used for the first time, but more commonly to something used for months or years. The rash persists for weeks or months. The allergy is lifelong.

Contact eczema is due to a 'delayed' allergic reaction. This means that the allergen may take 1-7 days (usually 2) to produce an allergic reaction. Testing for contact allergy is done by applying a 'battery' of allergens to the skin of the back (patch tests). They are applied under little metal discs held in place by tape for 48 hours. These are then removed and the back examined for reactions. The back is checked again at 5 days to make sure no other reactions have appeared. The reaction looks like eczema with redness and scaling or even blisters if severe.

The allergens routinely tested are nickel, other metals, preservatives, some antibiotics, primula, perfumes, rubber, chemicals and hair dye, and on occasion many other substances.

Common causes of this kind of skin allergy are:

Metal Allergy (nickel allergy). One in ten women suffers from this. It is a reaction to nickel which is present in most metals, especially those used in 'cheap' jewellery. Many women develop itchy ears from such earrings and solve the problem by changing to sterling silver or gold jewellery. Foreign silver, rolled gold and gold plating all contain nickel and cause the eczema to reappear (see illustration).

All such jewellery should be given away, otherwise the temptation to wear it is occasionally irresistible and itchy weeping ears result. The same problem arises from jeans studs, and a patch of eczema near the belly button is often caused by these. Watches, safety pins, bra clips and zips can all cause the same problem. Most women find this only a minor problem and change to different jewellery and watches. Sterling silver, high carat gold, platinum and stainless steel are nickel-free (but also more expensive!). In those that are sensitive all clothes, particularly bras, should be examined before buying to ensure that clips and zips are plastic. Covering clips and studs with paint, lacquer or nail varnish is a very unsatisfactory alternative. Persistent wearing of nickel can cause the rash to spread all over the body.

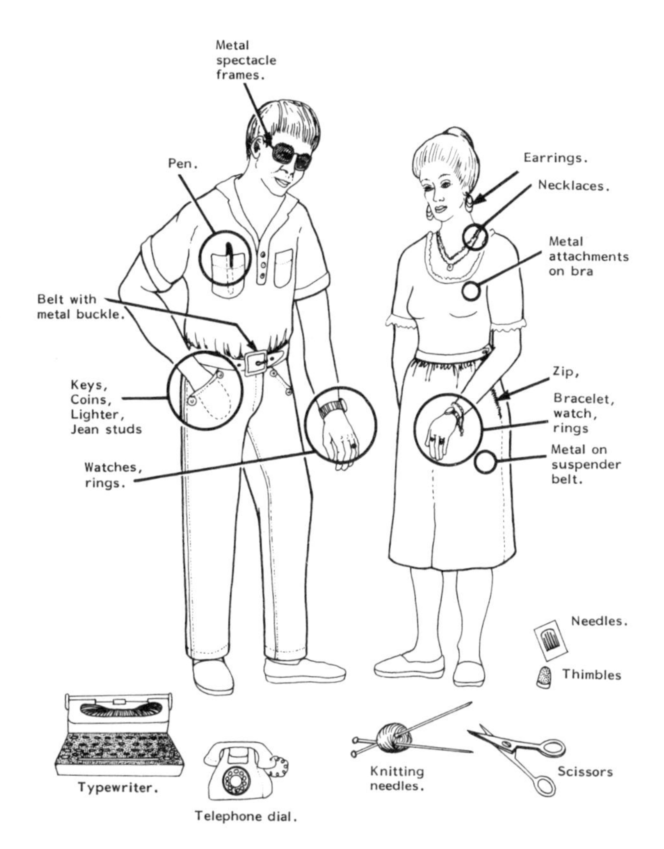

Perfume Allergy. There are many individual fragrance substances in perfumes which can cause allergy. Each one occurs in many different perfumes. This can be a great nuisance as most cosmetics, soaps and toiletries are perfumed. Other people's perfume sprays may trigger off the eczema.

Many people who know they are allergic to perfume switch to baby products, but those are also scented and the eczema continues.

A new problem for men is allergy to synthetic musk, a perfume in aftershaves. An eczema comes out on the face and sun-exposed sites (see Chapter 1) in strong sunlight. This musk is also present in some shaving creams, soaps, talc, deodorants, shampoos, hair creams, and baby products, so the rash persists even after abandoning aftershaves.

People with perfume allergy should use only products that specifically state that they are unscented, e.g. Simple brand, Almay, ROC, Clinique, Marks & Spencer's unperfumed cosmetics.

Cosmetic Allergies. All cosmetics contain potential allergens. The commonest are lanolin, perfumes and preservatives (which stop cosmetics going bad).

Cosmetic allergy usually causes a rash on the face, the very sensitive areas around the eyes being worst affected, becoming very swollen and itchy.

Nail varnish can cause contact eczema of the areas of skin touched by the finger nails, e.g. eyelids and neck, but the fingers are not affected. Almay and ROC nail varnish do not cause this problem.

Herbal cosmetics do not contain fewer allergens than conventional ones.

Hypoallergenic cosmetics can also cause allergies, as all compounds are potential allergens and they do contain lanolin and preservatives. However, they omit perfumes and other common allergens. Check with the manufacturers whether they contain lanolin before buying.

Hair dyes often cause problems, usually in people who have been dyeing their hair for years. The dye (paraphenylenediamine) causes itching and weeping of the forehead, neck and behind the ears. A severe reaction involves the whole face and extends on to the shoulders and the rest of the body. This is why hair dyeing preparations recommend a patch test before use. It is better to have an itchy patch on the arm than a face like a tomato.

Plant Allergy. The plants commonly causing allergy are primulas and chrysanthemums in Britain, and poison ivy in North America.

Very gentle and brief contact with the plant can cause severe skin reaction with swelling and blisters on the area touched and on the eyelids and face.

Medicament Allergy. Creams and ointments used for medical purposes can cause contact eczema. When this happens there is a marked worsening of the original skin problem. Anti-itch (antihistamine), local anaesthetic and antibiotic creams and eye drops are the chief offenders.

Rubber Allergy. Rubber gloves can cause an allergic rash over the backs of the hands, wrists and lower arms. This often occurs when people who already have a skin problem use rubber gloves to protect their broken skin. PVC gloves, Boots Long Life gloves and Glovelies should then be used.

Rubber shoes can also cause a reaction.

Coping with Contact Eczema

Avoid the allergen, and the rash will go away. The initial discomfort can be helped by steroid creams from your doctor. Often the cause of the allergy is not obvious and requires special patch tests done at a skin clinic to unravel the mystery.

Contact Urticaria (nettle rash)

This is rare. Some people react within minutes with weals to skin contact with certain foods, e.g. fish or eggs, animal fur and other compounds. This also happens when stung by a nettle.

Skin Reactions to Substances Taken Internally

Allergens from foods, medicines, stings and infections can enter the blood and cause the skin to react in the following ways:

Urticaria

Urticaria is also called nettle rash or hives. Areas of skin become itchy and raised into weals which are red or white. These persist for minutes or hours. In very severe attacks the eyelids, mouth and even throat can swell. If the throat and mouth swell, urgent hospital treatment is necessary.

Urticaria is usually *not* due to allergy, but because it seems so mysterious and inexplicable people always assume it is. They often make fruitless complex alterations to their diet and lifestyle, avoiding mythical allergens. This results in a miserable life in addition to an unpleasant skin rash.

In a minority of cases there is a cause for the urticaria. They are:

Foods may cause urticaria and usually the cause is obvious. Shellfish, nuts, strawberries or other fruits are the most common. Sometimes dyes or preservatives in foods can be the cause.

Drugs. Aspirin may cause urticaria or make it much worse. People often do not realise that it is present in headache and indigestion remedies, and take it unknowingly.
Penicillin and other antibiotics and drugs can also cause urticaria.
Physical Causes. Heat and cold (see Chapter 1), and sunlight can all cause urticaria.
Stings. Some unfortunate individuals develop urticaria in response to bee or wasp stings. This can be so severe that the mouth and throat swell.

These account for very few cases of urticaria. In most cases the cause is unknown.

Prick testing is used to find out the cause of urticaria. These tests are performed by pricking a drop of a test substance into the skin of the inner forearm. If there is a reaction a coloured swelling (weal) appears within 20 minutes. There is a standard battery of test substances containing extracts of milk, egg and other foods, pollens, house dust mites and animal fur. This reaction is an 'immediate type' of allergic reaction as it occurs within minutes, causes only a weal surrounded by a red flare and fades quickly. A similar process occurs in hayfever and asthma.

If a cause for the urticaria can be identified then it must always be scrupulously avoided. You will never lose the allergy. If the cause cannot be identified, then enough antihistamine tablets must be taken to suppress the urticaria until it goes away. This will usually entail increasing the number of tablets rather than changing to different types. They must be taken regularly to prevent the rash coming up, *not* after it has developed.

Antihistamine Tablets

Piriton (chloropheniramine)
Phenergan (promethazine)
Anthisan (mepyramine)
Vallergan (trimeprazine)

In a severe or unexpected urticarial reaction, you should take double your normal dose of antihistamine as soon as possible. The reaction may be very alarming, but will respond to tablets within 30-60 minutes and seldom needs injections.

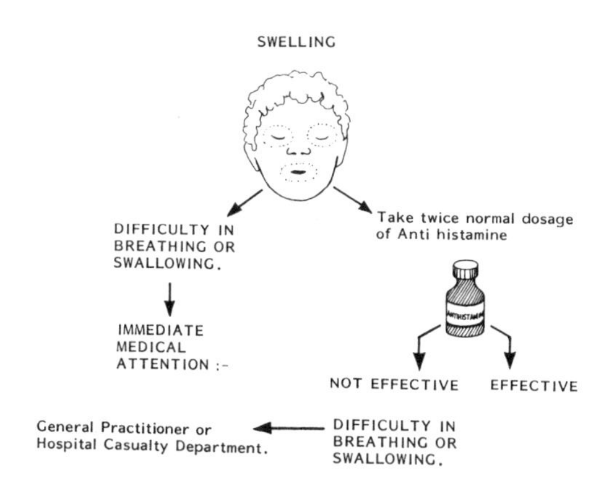

3. Common Skin Problems

Psoriasis

What is Psoriasis?

Psoriasis is a very common disease in Britain—it is estimated that 1-2 million people suffer from it. The main problem is that the skin grows too rapidly in some places, forming a silvery scale over thick patches which become inflamed and red.

Patches of psoriasis develop over areas where the skin is frequently knocked such as the elbows and knees, and it happens where the skin has been injured in grazes and cuts and operation scars. The scalp is badly affected and the scaling gives rise to hard lumps and very flaky dandruff. However, anywhere on the skin may be affected and some people have red scaly skin all over.

A small number of psoriasis sufferers have arthritis, especially of the finger and toe joints which become red, swollen and stiff. Nails also grow very fast and may be thick and flaky.

Psoriasis is harmless but can become very distressing as it can be very difficult to cope with the appearance of the skin. Many sufferers dislike exposing their skin when sunbathing or playing sports. In addition, painful fissures can be troublesome and itching can be a nuisance.

Is it Catching?

It is not possible to catch psoriasis. Most people start to get patches between the ages of 15 and 25 but it can develop at any age from childhood to extreme old age (I have seen a man who was 96 when he first developed the problem).

If you Have Inherited the Tendency to Psoriasis

It seems that psoriasis runs in families. Many people who have psoriasis will know relatives with psoriasis. Attacks may be triggered by an illness, especially a sore throat, an operation, the use of certain drugs, or injury to the skin (such as sunburn).

Will It Go Away?

Each patch of psoriasis tends to come and go over the years leaving perfectly normal looking skin. How often the patches come and go forms your own pattern of psoriasis and is impossible for anyone to predict.

Psoriasis tends to get better in summer (see below) and worse in winter, but tends to come and go on its own and may clear up completely for years before a new patch develops. However, once you have had psoriasis it is always possible for you to have psoriasis again. Many people have stubborn little patches on the elbows and knees that are almost permanent.

What Can Be Done About It?

This depends very much on how you feel about it—some people mind very little about having very bad psoriasis and find the treatments more trouble than the disease. No magic treatment will remove psoriasis once and for all—all treatments are aimed at slowing the growth of your skin and clearing up individual patches. If you are happy with your psoriasis—keep it—it won't do you any harm. If you want treatment there are many types available from your doctor.

Ointments. Most psoriasis treatments are ointments based on coal tar and dithranol. These can be very effective although they take some months to work. They are smelly and stain clothes and the skin so it is best to apply them at night and use old sheets. Dithranol can burn the skin so should be applied very carefully only to the psoriasis. Steroid ointments such as Dermovate and Betnovate when prescribed by your doctor may help for a short time, but the effect tends to wear off rapidly and the skin can get worse again if too much is used. A mild steroid cream (hydrocortisone) may help in the creases of the body where the skin is delicate and cannot tolerate coal tar.

Ultraviolet Light (see Chapter 1). Ultraviolet radiation from sunshine, for example 2-3 weeks sunbathing, may clear your psoriasis for some months. Ultraviolet lamps will also clear the psoriasis and may be helpful in 4-6 week courses but should be used longer only on your doctor's advice as prolonged treatment may give harmful long-term effects (see Chapter 1). Sunburn must be avoided as this will worsen the psoriasis. Sunbeds and ultraviolet A (UVA) lamps will only really improve the psoriasis if used in combination with drugs called Psoralens (UVA treatment). Regular PUVA treatment will usually control bad psoriasis but increases the risk of skin aging and skin cancer, especially in fair skin. This treatment is used only for bad psoriasis and under medical supervision.

Drugs by Mouth. Many of the anti-cancer drugs will slow down skin growth and control psoriasis. However, they usually have unpleasant side effects. Methotrexate is used in very severe psoriasis and has to be taken continuously. Regular liver and blood checks are essential. New drugs derived from vitamin A (Retinoids) have been used for psoriasis but they also cause liver and blood problems (with raised blood fats) and are used only in severe cases.

As yet, there is no easy and safe cure for psoriasis. A lot of help can be gained by talking to other people and learning how they cope with their psoriasis. The Psoriasis Association has a regular newsletter and meetings but if they don't live near you, why not start your own support group by advertising locally? It is surprising how often psoriasis seems to improve when you come to terms with it.

Living with Psoriasis

'I am 14 and have had psoriasis for about 7 years. I think being in my teens it's twice as hard to accept. I never used to wear fashionable clothes or anything above my knees. My arms had to be covered and I had to have a long fringe to cover my forehead. In the last few months during the summer holidays I told myself that I had psoriasis, a skin condition which will stay with me for life. I gave myself a choice. Feel sorry for yourself, hide away and allow yourself to believe the childish things you're called. Or accept that you have, for some reason, got psoriasis and it won't go away. So make the best of your life and live. I took the second choice and started wearing the modern clothes that I'd seen so many people wear, I bought expensive clothes and the cheap clothes in the market like ra-ras that mum had asked if I wanted in June. Then I'd said "I can't wear them", or "It'll show my spots". I stopped being jealous of my 11-year-old sister who didn't have psoriasis and wore anything. I think the reason for my psoriasis going down is that I'm not so het up and I think people aren't always staring. I think psoriasis affects you inwardly so that's why it's at its worst if you are depressed.

Now, because I've changed my attitude to life, people don't call me names or talk about me behind my back. It's not so hush-hush any more. Believing in myself has also changed my vocabulary so that if someone says, "Er, what's that?" I say, "Oh, it's just a skin trouble or skin irritation" because I think "skin disease" sounds awful. But I still remember one thing about being called names that hurt, really hurt. When my friend, my best friend, was asking around for plimsolls to borrow for a netball match I lent her mine and I was walking up stairs after P.E. when people were changing, and a girl said to my best friend, "Oh don't wear them, she's got a contagious disease". Just as she said this I stepped into the room. I could have sunk into the floor, I wished the world would gobble me up, but I thought this is your chance. Tell them, I thought, and I did. "It's not contagious, and anyone saying different can go and see the headmistress". That shut them up.

So remember if you feel good inside you'll look good outside and you'll be buying minis and bikinis in bulk!'

(from 'Beyond the Ointment',
the journal of the Psoriasis Association)

Useful Address:

The Psoriasis Association,
7 Milton Street,
Northampton NN2 7JG.
Tel. 0604 711129

Acne

Acne is very common in the teens and twenties. A plague of pimples appears at a time when looking your best may seem so important.

The Cause

Acne is not caused by germs or dirt. The male sex hormones (androgens) cause acne. At puberty in boys the androgens cause the voice to break, beard to grow, the skin to become greasy and spots to erupt.

All women have both female hormones (oestrogen and progesterone) and androgens. Acne is due to an imbalance of these hormones and not to extra male hormones. Greasy skin, excess facial and body hair, and the thinning of scalp hair can also be due to this imbalance.

Pregnancy improves acne because of the large amounts of female hormones secreted at this time.

Who Gets Acne?

All teenagers have some acne, varying from a few blackheads to a very unsightly and upsetting problem with large red lumps and cysts and large pus-filled spots. Most people grow out of acne in their twenties, some as late as the thirties.

In most women changes in the balance of female hormones at period time causes a few acne spots each month. The oral contraceptive pill may either improve acne or make it worse.

Where Do You Get Acne?

Acne affects the face, usually the forehead, cheeks and chin. The 'beard area' is often the worst affected in older women.

The shoulders, back and chest are often involved, and may be much worse than the face.

How Do Spots Form?

The blackheads, spots and lumps of acne are all related to the grease (sebaceous) glands. The gland produces grease (sebum) which drains on to the skin. The opening is visible as a 'pore'.

Androgens increase the amount of grease formed and block the opening of the gland. The blockage is visible as a blackhead and the gland becomes swollen and inflamed (see Diagram), with swelling and redness which you see as a spot. If severe, it forms large painful deep cysts.

The pore may also be blocked by heavy greasy makeup, hair products, moisturisers and suntan oils, and sometimes by hot, sweaty conditions.

Myths About Acne

Acne is *not* due to dirt or an infection.

There is no scientific evidence that your diet affects acne.

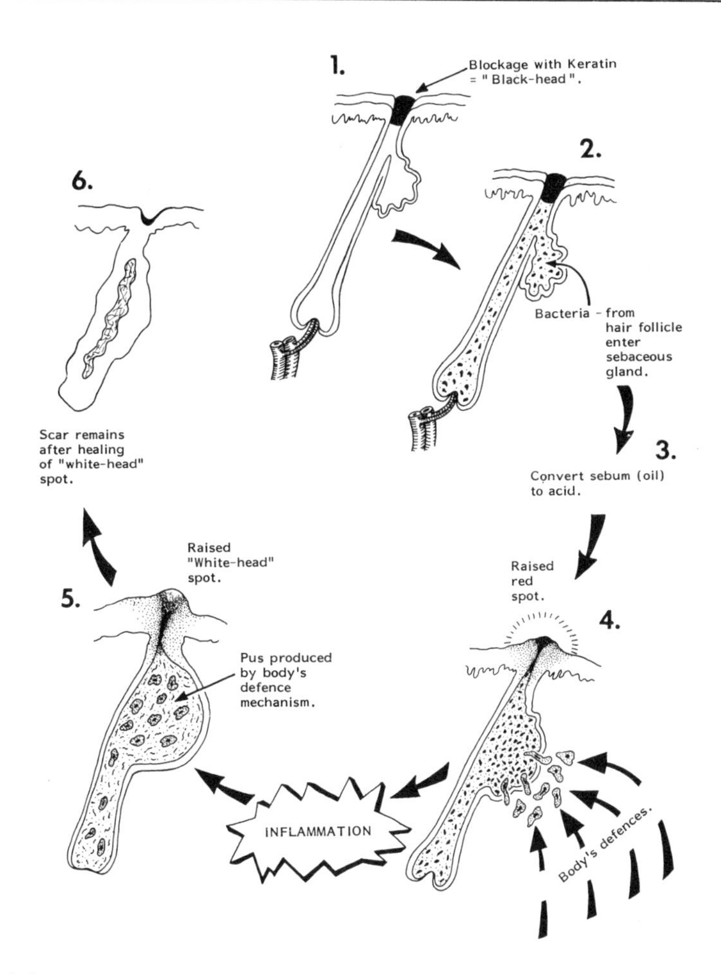

Many people cut out greasy foods and chocolates but only a few benefit.

Life with acne is miserable enough without worrying if you've inflicted it on yourself by either 'dirtiness' or your diet.

How to Treat Acne

Acne can be treated very successfully. Bad acne needs a doctor's help early, before you have become depressed and discouraged by no benefit from over-the-counter acne preparations.

You cannot wash away acne. Washing will only temporarily remove the grease, which will soon be replaced. Some special washes and cleansers may even make blackheads worse.

Preparations to Put on the Skin

There is a vast and bewildering array of preparations for acne—lotions, gels, creams, ointments, scrubs and soaps. Many are of slight benefit, some harmful.

Peeling Agents

Peeling of the skin unblocks the pores which helps blackheads and small spots.

Face masks, light peeling (in beauty salons), abrasive scrubs and sponges all work in this way but the effects are shortlived. Most acne preparations are peeling agents and the most effective contain benzoyl peroxide. Preparations containing other ingredients, e.g. resorcinol, sulphur, antiseptics, are not as good so check the ingredients before you buy.

Antibiotics

Antibiotic lotions containing clindamycin or erythromycin (from a doctor) are successful in treating acne but take about two months to work. Other antibiotic lotions are probably useless.

Retinoic Acid

Retinoic acid (from vitamin A) from your doctor, put on the skin, slowly clears blackheads. The disadvantages are peeling and drying, and darkening of black skin.

Steroids

Steroid creams, such as Betnovate, Synalar and Dermovate, must NEVER be put on acne as they make it worse in the long run even if they help temporarily.

Steroid injections (by a doctor) can help to heal large painful cysts.

Acne Preparations

containing sulphur

Dome-Acne
Actinac
Eskamel
Neomedrone

containing benzoyl peroxide

Acnegel
Benoxyl
Panoxyl
Acetoxyl
Quinoderm

peeling agents

Brasivol
Ionax

Sun Lamps and Sunlight

Sunlight usually improves acne. Suntan oils prevent the benefit of sunshine by blocking pores, so should not be used.

Artificial sun lamps or UVA lamps are not as helpful. The tan disguises some of the redness and makes the acne look better.

Make-up

Non-greasy make-up can be worn and is often helpful in hiding the spots.

Thick heavy make-up, moisturisers or cleansers will make acne worse and must be avoided. There is a wide range of make-up for acne sufferers, usually advertised as oil-free or for oily/greasy skin.

Preparations to take by mouth

Tablets are required for all moderate or severe cases of acne.

All tablets take two to three months to work. Many people get fed up during the first few weeks and do not take them for long enough.

Antibiotics are very effective. They suppress the inflammation of the acne spots and cut down skin bacteria. Tetracyclines are most commonly used. Erythromycin and septrin can be used, but other antibiotics do not work.

Antibiotics are taken in very long courses, usually nine months or more. The acne clears in two to six months and then the antibiotic is slowly reduced every three months or so. Many people need one tablet a day or less for years to keep the skin clear. There are no long-term side-effects from this.

Hormone Treatment

The anti-androgen Cyproterone (combined with oestrogen in Diane) is a new experimental treatment for women. It stops the skin and hair being greasy and clears the spots. Men need their male hormones and cannot take this treatment.

The Pill and Acne

The Pill contains varying amounts of oestrogen and progestogens. Some pills containing more or stronger progestogens will make acne worse. A few will improve acne.

If you have acne, or acne starts while you are on the Pill, discuss with your doctor which pill will be most helpful.

Will Acne Leave Scars?

Everyone worries about scarring, but it is rare. The scarring depends on your type of skin. Early and effective treatment from your doctor will mean less scarring. The chest and back scar more often than the face. It is doubtful whether picking and squeezing makes much difference. The types of scars are small 'ice pick' scars (tiny pits), large pits and raised lumpy scars (keloids) (see Chapter 5).

Spots leave red or dark marks and these disappear within months. Nothing makes them disappear any faster.

Treatment of Scars

There are an unfortunate few who do get scars. The pits will improve with the years, or collagen injections can sometimes be helpful (see Chapter 5).

How to Live With Your Acne

If you have acne be optimistic. It is not a life sentence and it can be controlled while you grow out of it. A new spot before an important date seems like a major disaster, but don't cancel the outing—cover up the spot. Remember your spots seem bigger, redder and more numerous to you than to anyone else.

Use ordinary soap to wash your skin and a peeling agent for the blackheads. Get outside into the sunlight. Eat a normal diet. Wear make-up if you wish, but avoid greasy and oily cosmetics. An acne treatment at a beauty salon can produce a good temporary improvement before an important event.

If you have bad acne your doctor or the skin specialist will help but it takes several months.

An Acne Sufferer's Experience

'I have now been suffering from acne for about seven years and it didn't start until I was eighteen. Like any illness only those who have suffered from this particular skin complaint can actually know of the soreness, pain and the self-consciousness and embarrassment it carries. When it flares up very badly it is red and inflamed and then extremely sore and uncomfortable. If it gets knocked or it bleeds it is very painful. From my personal experience it has affected certain areas on my face and on the back and chest. It sometimes calms down for a while but then flares up again, usually in the same areas. Although many people are left with scars, I find that once a patch dies down the redness does disappear, although this can take some considerable time.

Apart from the pain one suffers, every acne sufferer is so conscious of the fact it is there. Everyone will notice it and you must be very strong and confident not to let this worry you but to try to ignore it. You have to get used to it, be confident that it will be cured and, although difficult, do not let it affect your everyday life. Many people will mention it to you and often it is difficult to accept they are only trying to help you. I have found that those close to you who see you every day tend to get accustomed to it, but socially I am always extremely conscious of it. However, although acne is a very painful complaint you must hope that with time it will heal, while there are thousands of people with permanent facial scars or disabilities whose problems never will.'

Infections

Skin infections can come back again and again. Knowing more about them helps to come to terms with the attacks.

Herpes

There are two herpes viruses—herpes simplex virus which causes cold sores and genital herpes and another virus which causes chickenpox.

Cold Sores

Most people get cold sores in childhood from someone with a cold sore. The first attack is the worst. Small children may get painful mouth ulcers and swollen glands. Usually, a group of small blisters appears on the lips, forms a crust and dries up after seven to ten days. The virus then becomes dormant in the nerve and can be reactivated by illness and high fevers, especially colds and sore throats, and by sunshine. Cold sores come back in the same place.

Coping with Cold Sores. The dormant virus cannot be removed from the nerves by any method. During an attack antiseptic lotions (Betadine, surgical spirit) dry up the blisters and prevent other germs prolonging the cold sore. Idoxuridine lotion (Herpid) and acyclovir (Zovirax) cream are antivirus treatments your doctor may prescribe for very bad cases. If you are prone to repeated cold sores use a sun blocking preparation when sunbathing, climbing mountains or skiing. There are now also lip screens available, e.g. Roc.

Genital Herpes

This is caused by a different strain of the same virus, caught by having sex with someone who has herpes. It is common in young people. Groups of little blisters appear on the genital area, thighs and buttocks. They are painful, tender and highly infectious. The first infection is the worst with swollen glands and a temperature. The blisters crust over and clear in seven to ten days. The virus becomes dormant but may cause repeated attacks.

Coping with Genital Herpes. The virus (hidden in the nerves) cannot be killed. Antiviral creams and lotions, used immediately, may shorten an attack. Warm salt water baths and painkillers (aspirin or paracetamol) make you more comfortable during an attack. All attacks of genital herpes are infectious to your lover.

You should not have sex during an attack but once the scabs have disappeared, you can have sex again. Condoms lessen the risk of infection.

An attack of genital herpes in pregnancy is very serious as an infected mother can pass on the infection to her baby and so she may need to be delivered by a caesarean section.

Frequent attacks play havoc with your sex life. New vaccines and antiviral drugs are being developed which hold some hope. Worry and depression, poor general health or lack of sleep and an unhealthy diet may reduce your resistance to infection.

Genital herpes is in the news and people have been frightened by speculations in the press. Although repeated herpes can be a big problem, many people only have a single mild attack.

Shingles

After chickenpox, the virus lives in the nerves. Later in life, very painful crops of blisters (the Danish call it 'a belt of roses from hell') may appear in the skin on one side of the body supplied by the nerve. They last 7-14 days. Most people have only one attack of shingles. Painkillers help the pain, which is usually worst as the attack is developing, but sometimes comes on for weeks or months after the blisters have gone. Seek your doctor's advice immediately for shingles on the face (the blisters are confined to one side of the face) as it can damage the eyes.

Aids Virus (H.T.L.V. III)

AIDS (Acquired immune deficiency syndrome) virus depresses immunity, increasing the risk of common and rare infections and rare cancers (particularly Kaposi's sarcoma). Although this is commoner in homosexual males, it may be transmitted heterosexually or by infected blood products. Kaposi's sarcoma shows as purple lumps and patches on the skin. Although rubber gloves and condoms are reported as reducing risk of infection there is no evidence for this.

Warts

There are several strains of wart virus causing warts in different places. You may have thick hard warts on the soles of the feet (verrucae); cauliflower-like warts on the hands, face and knees; flat warts on the face; or genital warts.

Children catch the wart virus at school from someone else's wart. After three to four months the warts appear. The body's defences work very slowly against the warts so they last a very long time, usually about two years but sometimes up to ten years. Eventually, the body kills the wart virus and the wart drops off, often very suddenly (explaining some miracle cures).

Genital Warts are transmitted by contact in the sexually active. Other diseases may be caught at the same time. They may be related to the development of cervical cancer so if you have warts, get them treated properly and have regular cervical smears.

Coping with Warts. Although warts are infectious, preventing children from swimming when they have warts is unnecessary. (Plastic protective socks (Plastsox) can be worn if the school insists.) As most people get warts, it is better to have your warts as a child than as an adult, when they will be more unsightly and troublesome. Once you have had warts you will be resistant to them as an adult.

No treatment can kill the wart virus. The wart will disappear on its own. Most treatments are hard skin removers which peel the top off the wart in the hope that the body will kill the virus (e.g. Salactol). More dramatic treatments include scraping, burning or freezing the warts. These physically destroy the wart but it often comes back and unpleasant scars can result. Remember—untreated, the wart would disappear without trace. Wart charming, selling the wart to a friend, hypnosis or dandelion juice at midnight have much to recommend them—they are painless, harmless and leave no scars. If warts are painful to walk on, corn plasters (20% salicylic acid plasters) will soften the hard skin.

Wart Preparations from the chemist

(Caution—avoid normal skin)

Peeling agents (also for corns)

Salicylic acid plasters (20%, 40%)
Salicylic acid collodion
Salactol (salicylic acid and lactic acid)
Duofilm (,, ,,)

Other agents

Glutaraldehyde (Glutarol, Verucasept)
Formalin (Veracur)

Podophylin paint/Posalfilin should not be used.

Boils

Infection of hair roots with bacteria (staphylococci) causes boils. Repeated attacks are common in teenagers and young adults. A red painful lump will develop a head of pus which bursts and leaves a scar. Courses of antibiotics may clear single attacks of boils. People who have repeated attacks may need intensive skin disinfection. To clear the germ from the nose, the armpits and groin, you need a nasal antiseptic cream and antiseptic bath solution such as Hibiscrub or Betadine. Do not use Savlon or Dettol baths as these may harm your skin.

Athlete's Foot

Athlete's foot is caused by a fungus which grows in the soggy toe spaces of sweaty or unwashed feet. Plastic or rubber shoes and dirty socks encourage this. The infection causes itching, redness and blistering which may spread to the groin. Elsewhere on the body it forms the rings of ringworm. Ringworm is common in tropical parts of the world.

Coping with Athlete's Foot. Wear cotton socks, open sandals and powder the toe spaces. Antifungal creams and powders will help and may need to be used for a very long time.

Antifungus preparations

From the Chemist (not effective against thrush)
Whitfield's ointment (Compound benzoic acid ointment)
Tineaderm—cream, lotion, powder (Tolnaftate)
Mycota—cream, spray, dusting powder (Zinc undecenoate)
Tineafax—powder, ointment

Thrush (Candida)

Thrush can cause sores at the angles of the mouth, especially in false teeth wearers where it lurks above the dental plate. Babies may get white patches of thrush on the tongue and sides of the mouth.

Thrush infection of the vagina with itching and discharge is common and many women have thrush in several places at once.

Having the hands frequently immersed in water (hard to avoid for barmaids, washers-up, domestic workers, housewives) and pushing the cuticles back can cause redness and swelling around the finger nails due to thrush infection.

Coping with Thrush. To help stop the nail problems, avoid water by wearing rubber or plastic gloves. Also, do not push cuticles back. For mouth problems, wear better fitting false teeth, take them out at night and scrub the dentures well with a nailbrush.

Vaginal thrush usually clears with pessaries such as Nystatin and clotrimazole. The contraceptive pill, antibiotics and pregnancy can create conditions which encourage thrush. Prolonged use of pessaries may help. Women's health groups suggest applying natural live yoghurt which contains harmless bacteria to replace the thrush. Avoid nylon panty tights and tight jeans as a warm, moist environment encourages thrush to grow.

Pityriasis Versicolor

(also known as Tinea Versicolor)

This very common skin problem is a superficial fungus which stops the skin tanning. Most people discover the infection on holiday as they get small, round, white patches on the back and chest. If you are not tanned the patches may be reddish-brown. Heat and humidity encourage the infection.

Coping with Pityriasis Versicolor. Diluted Selsun shampoo (equal parts with water) can be used as a lotion on the trunk and scalp. Two overnight applications will be enough. The colour takes months to return and often needs more sunshine. Do not keep using the treatment as this will dry out your skin.

Nits *(Lice on the scalp)*

Nits cause havoc in schools. The adult lice run from one scalp to another, sticking eggs on to the hairs with a strong cement-like substance. The pearly nits look like sticky dandruff, but cannot be shaken off. Running a nail along the hair will not detach the eggs.

Dealing with Nits. Anti-louse lotion, either gamma benzene hexachloride lotion or cream (Lorexane, Gammexane) or malathion (Prioderm), will kill the eggs which can be removed by a comb with very fine teeth. One treatment is enough but all the family who are infested should be treated, and the hair examined regularly for a while. If many school children have lice, the whole school must be examined to prevent repeated attacks.

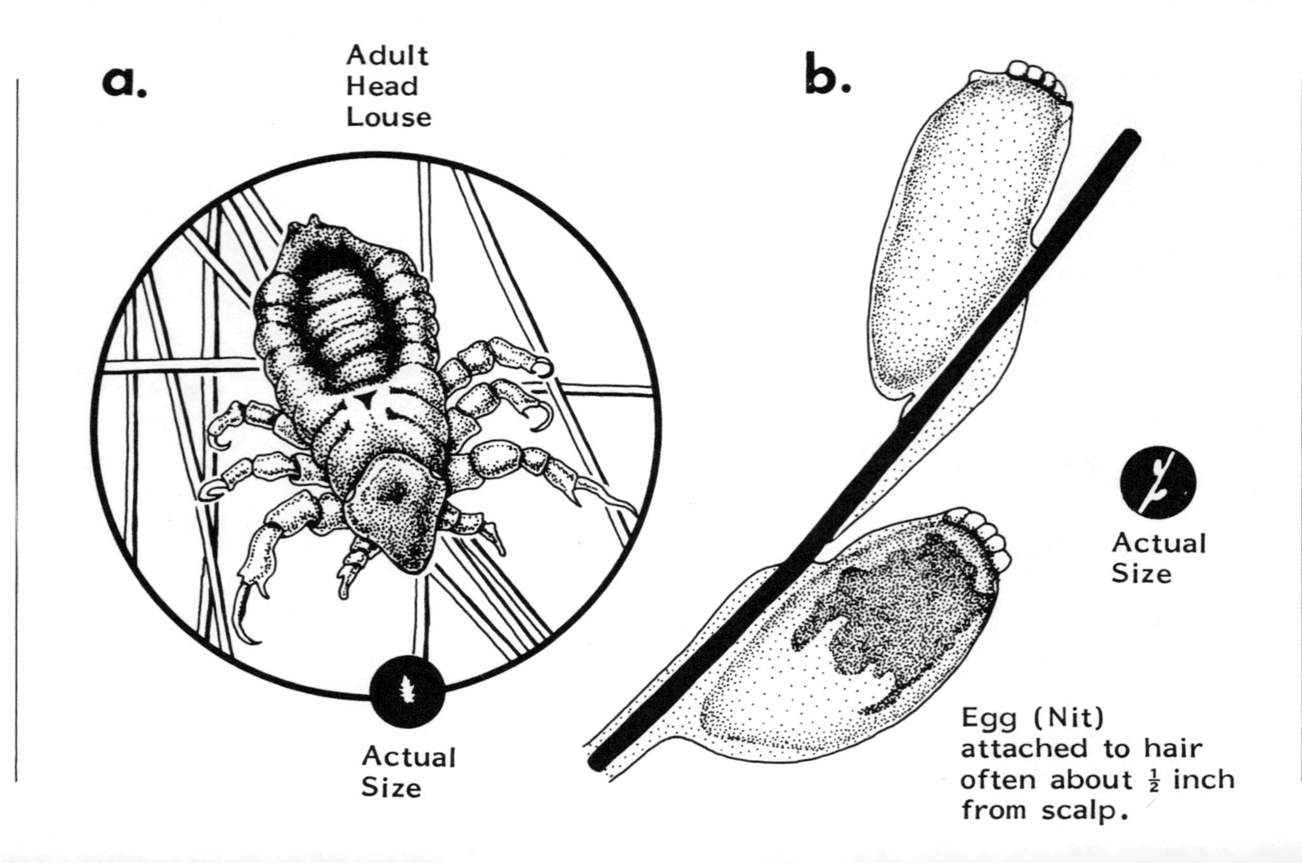
a.
Adult
Head
Louse
Actual
Size
b.
Actual
Size
Egg (Nit)
attached to hair
often about ½ inch
from scalp.

Insect Bites

Many people get bitten by insects. We usually know if we have been bitten by mosquitoes, wasps or bees. Only a few people are allergic to bites from less obvious insects and get itchy lumps from them. The bites are often in groups or lines and last for weeks. They may blister—like chickenpox—but are usually worst on the legs. Old bites will start itching in sympathy with new bites. The source of the insects, usually fleas or mites, is often from domestic pets. Less often, the house is infested with fleas, bed bugs or mites (tiny insects that you can't see). Rats or mice can carry insects into old buildings. You may never see the insects. You will have to treat the source of the insects to stop the bites, rather than putting anything on your skin.

Preventing Insect Bites. First you should disinfest your pet every week with a spray or shampoo from the vet or pet shop. Flea collars are not enough. Change and spray the animal's bedding frequently. Do not get rid of your pet as you will get more bites rather than fewer. New fleas hatch in the carpets for years and will bite you if there is no cat or dog. Remember, someone else's dog or cat may be to blame. Vapona Insecticide strips in affected rooms also kill fleas.

If you have thoroughly treated your pets and household, and the problem is not getting better, get the advice of your public health department—the address is in the post office or phone book.

4. Hair

Facts About Normal Hair

We can change our looks drastically by styling, curling, bleaching and straightening our hair. A multi-million pound industry is based on persuading us that this is essential for our attractiveness.

The Structure of Hair

The hair that we see above the scalp is dead hair and the growing area (hair bulb) is deeply embedded in the scalp below the surface. Each hair has its own grease gland. The core of hair contains the colour pigment which is lacking in grey hair. The cuticle is the hard outside of the hair and is made of overlapping scales. The number of hair roots on the scalp is about 100,000.

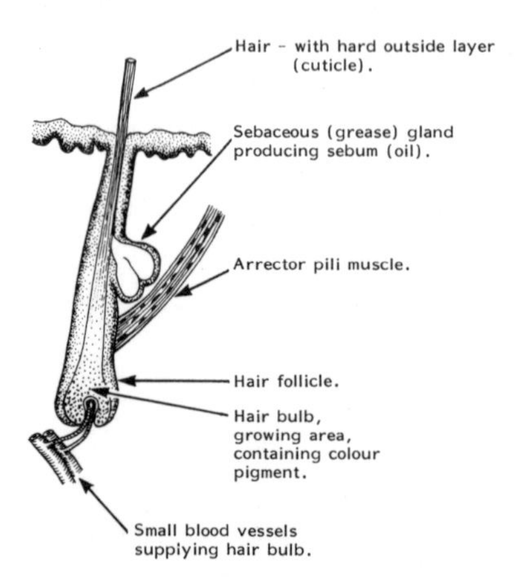

The Life of a Hair

Each root grows many hairs in a lifetime. Every hair grows for about 1000 days and rests for 100 days before it falls out by a dying-back of the root releasing it from the scalp. It is replaced by a new hair from the same root. We lose about 100 hairs a day.

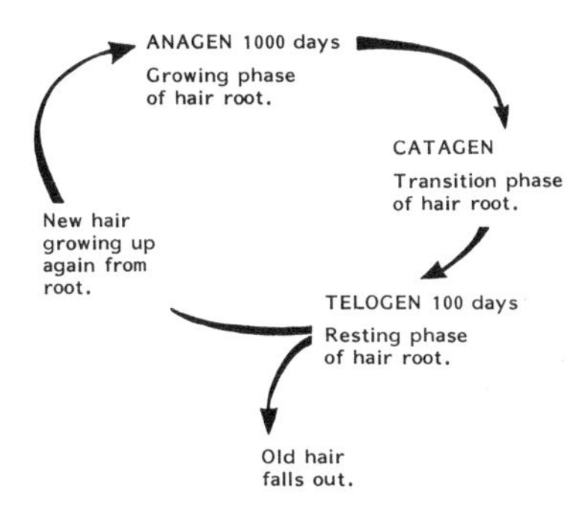

Curly or Straight

The curl of hair depends on genes inherited from your parents. Very curly hair is strongly inherited. The shape of the hair root decides whether hair is straight or curly as the hair grows asymmetrically within the root. The cross-section of the shape is round in straight hair and flattened in curly hair. The shape of hair can be altered by perming or straightening, but the way the hair grows cannot be altered.

Greasy or Dry

The oil from grease glands coats the hair. Overactive grease glands result in greasy hair but if grease glands are underactive the hair is dry and brittle. Shampooing does not alter the amount of grease produced by the gland. Greasy hair can be washed frequently and will be protected from damage by its coating.

Long Hair

Hair grows a few millimetres a day. There is a maximum length to which hair grows before it falls out. In most of us hair is as long as it ever will be after three years. In a few people, the hair grows fast or for longer than three years and is spectacularly long (Lady Godiva, Rapunzel). Cutting the hair won't make it grow faster but long hair gets straggly with split ends and cutting the ends makes it look thicker.

Thick or Thin Hair
The thickness of the hair varies with age and hormones. Some people have thin, fine hair and others coarse, thick, springy hair. If you lose hairs, the hair looks thinner.

'Weathering'
As the hair grows the cuticle becomes roughened and weathered. Weathering is the result of all the things you do to your hair including brushing and combing. Singeing is further damage. The hair breaks and the ends split. There is no way of glueing split ends together. Cut them off to prevent them splitting further.

Dandruff
The scalp is constantly growing and sheds the dead skin as scales. Excess shedding of normal scales is perceived as a problem in 5-10% of the population. Inflammation of the scalp, in seborrhoeic dermatitis or psoriasis (see Chapter 3), increases the scaling and dandruff. Normally frequent washing with anti-dandruff shampoos will control dandruff (see Chapter 2). If the scalp is itchy or red, creams from the doctor may be needed.

What we do to Hair

Change in Colour
Bleaching. Hydrogen peroxide takes the colour out of the hair. The bleaching is increased by ammonium persulphate. Some home kits contain both. Any bleaching causes the hair to become drier and more brittle.

Dyeing. Dyes can either coat the surface of the hair or penetrate the centre of the hair. Vegetable dyes such as henna (red) and chamomile (yellow) are used in shampoos and hair rinses, as well as dyes. They coat the surface of the hair and last through many shampoos.

Colour rinses attach themselves to the surface of the hair and are very easily washed out. They are available as shampoos.

Semipermanent dyes partially penetrate the hair and are retained for five to ten shampoos. They are a blend of red, yellow and blue dyes, and can give unpredictable colours on hair that has been permed or bleached. You may end up with a punk colour without meaning to!

Permanent dyes are the most commonly used. The dyes (related to paraphenylene diamine) penetrate into the centre of the hair where they cannot be removed by washing. To lighten dark hair bleaching has to happen first. Although all dyes can produce allergic reactions (see Chapter 2), the permanent dyes are the commonest causes of these reactions and then cannot be used again. All hair preparations contain perfumes and preservatives which can also cause allergies on the face and scalp.

Colour restorers are applied regularly over a long period to grey hair. They are metallic dyes (often lead). They need to be applied frequently as they build up on the surface. Anxiety about their lead content has restricted sales because of worries about lead poisoning. There is no real evidence of lead toxicity.

Change in Shape

Perming. A solution of ammonium thioglycollate breaks the chemical structure of the hair, softening it. The hair is wound on to curlers to form the curl and left for ten to forty minutes. The chemical structure is restored with a neutraliser. Overperming, perming bleached or coloured hair, or a mistake in the perm weakens the hair and it breaks off over the next few days to weeks.

Hair Straightening. The same chemicals as in hair perming are used but the hair is kept straight whilst forming the new shape.

Heat is also used to soften the hair or make it straight (hot combing or ironing).

Hair Cosmetics

Shampoos must remove grease, scales and dirt from the hair surface but must not be too efficient as hair completely free of oil is dull and lifeless and builds up static electricity. 20-30 years ago soaps were the basis of shampoos, but in hard water lime salts (scum) formed a dull coating to the hair which had to be removed by acid rinses (vinegar, lemon). Using soap instead of shampoos now will have a similar effect. Soaps have been replaced by anionic detergents based on sodium lauryl sulphate. These may be irritant to the eyes. Washing-up liquid is a suitable detergent but being efficient may remove too much grease and leave the hair dull. It may be used for very greasy hair. Grease is secreted on to the hair immediately after shampooing from between skin scales. Cleanliness is not related to foam formation but because of consumer demand, foam stabilisers are added. Other additives include lubricants—lanolin and proteins, anti-dandruff agents—selenum sulphide, zinc pyrithione and coal tar and preservatives. Shampoos are not in contact with the scalp for long enough to have much effect—they have little benefit in skin disease and seldom cause allergies on the scalp.

Hair conditioners were developed to reduce the static electricity which fluffs out the hair after shampooing and makes it difficult to comb. They coat the surface of the hair and may build up a thick layer—especially in fine blond hair which makes the hair limp. They are electrically charged dispersers of quaternary ammonium compounds (such as stearalkonium ammonium chloride) so when passed through the hair, static electricity is discharged attracting a fatty layer on to the hair shaft. These compounds are also irritating to the eyes. Animal proteins such as gelatin are added to thicken the coating layer and add 'body'.

Hair sprays form a plastic coating film around hairs to hold them in place. Shellac (resinous secretion of insects) was initially used but has been replaced by synthetic resins which are less brittle. Hair setting lotions are also gums or resins to coat the hair.

Hair tonics and restorers are ineffective compounds which irritate the scalp convincing the unfortunate user of their efficiency. Alas no hairs will grow, but you may develop a good dermatitis! Constituents include quinine, cantharides, oil of Cade, resorcin or sulphur.

All hair cosmetics contain perfumes and preservatives which may produce allergies on face, neck and ears.

Hair Problems — Too Little and Too Much

Severe hair problems may cause anguish. An increase in the number of hairs lost daily above about 200 hairs a day will be noticeable to the owner of the hair, who may become desperately anxious that he or she is going to become bald. This is usually not so, and the hair loss is not obvious to an outside observer, but the anguish caused by this is obviously worsened by the emphasis on hair appearance in advertisements and magazines.

Women may also be very worried by the growth of coarse dark hair in the wrong place—on the upper lips and chest, for example. Men seldom complain of too much hair, so this is not a problem for them.

Damaged Hair

Perming, straightening, hair dyeing and bleaching, hot combing, heated rollers, curling tongs and hot wax inevitably damage the hair. Dry brittle hair with split ends is a sign of this damage and if severe the hair will break. Tight braiding (cane rows) and pony tails will pull out the hair roots. Sunshine bleaches and dries hair.

Broken hairs with scaling can be caused by ringworm infection in children. Worried and unhappy children fiddle with and break off hair although the scalp itself is normal.

Coping with Damaged Hair. Do not colour permed hair and vice versa. Do not perm until the previously permed hair has completely grown out. Avoid overbrushing and tight spiky rollers. Use regular hair conditioners to counteract dryness—those containing lanolin are best. Avoid heated rollers, irons and curling tongs as well as hairdryers and vigorous towelling. Badly damaged hair breaks near the scalp. It is best to have a short hair style until the damaged hair has grown out. Do not wear tight braids or plaits.

Problems with Very Curly Hair

Very curly hair may curl into the scalp or beard, causing pus-filled spots. In black men, keloid scars may replace the spots (see Chapter 5). Close shaving will make the spots worse so grow a beard and wear the hair longer. Clipping or depilatory creams are preferable to shaving. Antiseptic cleansing lotions (Hibiscrub, Betadine, Savlon) reduce infection. If the spots persist see your doctor as antibiotics may help prevent the unsightly (and permanent) scars.

'Bald on Top'

Male baldness runs in families and is due to male hormones (androgens). It starts after puberty over the temples and hairline which recede, giving a high forehead. The top of the scalp loses all the hair and becomes smooth. Other men in the family—father, brother, uncle—are usually bald as well.

All women lose some hair as they grow older. Sometimes, the hair becomes fine and sparse over the front of the scalp from the teens onwards. Fortunately, in women, the loss is not usually complete. It is more noticeable to the sufferer than to anyone else. A change in hair style may provide excellent camouflage.

Coping with Baldness. There have been numerous potions and rituals to cure male baldness throughout history but none works. Nothing that is applied to the scalp can make hair roots grow. The only prevention for the male is castration before puberty which has unacceptable side effects!

In women, hormone treatment slows balding but may have long-term risks. Hair transplants are seldom necessary. Shortage of iron increases hair loss so if you have heavy periods, see your doctor in case you need iron tablets. Trichology cannot influence baldness, so don't waste your money.

Patchy Baldness (Alopecia areata)

The sudden appearance of small bald circles on the scalp or beard may seem like a world-shattering event. It is even more alarming if they grow larger and join up. The edge of the shiny smooth patch has tiny broken hairs. The baldness can follow an emotional upset but is quite common in healthy children and young people. Fortunately, these patches nearly always regrow after 6-12 months without any treatment. The new hair is often white but later becomes the normal colour. Complete baldness *(alopecia totalis)* is very rare. Many new treatments have been hailed as a breakthrough but all have been disappointing. Steroid tablets will produce temporary regrowth but the hair falls out. Local injections of steroids and strong steroid applications may accelerate regrowth but to do so may cause thinning and pitting of the scalp. Producing an allergic eczema on the scalp, using chemicals or plant extracts, may work, but they have to produce a severe eczema. Research is going on for a solution. Meanwhile, wigs can be provided by the NHS.

Temporary Baldness

Hair may suddenly fall out a few months after a serious illness or operation. Almost every woman loses some hair about three months after having a baby. Hairs shift from resting to growing during pregnancy and after the baby is delivered they go back to resting. Once the new hair starts to grow (after about three months) the old hairs are pushed out. So the hair loss is a sign that the new hair is on its way. The hair will remain thin until the new hair grows out and if you have long hair it may be twelve to eighteen months before it looks normal. There is nothing your doctor can do as long as you are now well in yourself. Perming helps to disguise the loss.

'I Look Like a Man'

Facial Hair. Coarse dark hair on the upper lip and beard area affects 30% of young women. This is more noticeable in brunettes and is due to the effects of certain hormones.

Coarse Body Hair. Dark hair on the body may be very noticeable on legs, upper thighs and arms, and may grow around the nipples, on the chest and in the navel.

Coping with Excess Hair. Waxing, bleaching, shaving, plucking and depilatory creams will all remove the visible hair but do not reduce the growth from the root. They have no side effects, are safe on the face and may be used for years. They do *not* make the hair grow faster or coarser, contrary to popular belief. The new hairs feel coarser because they are all the same length. Bleaching will make the hair less noticeable.

Electrolysis is the only permanent way of stopping the hair from growing—an electrode is passed down each individual hair and the root is destroyed. Sometimes electrolysis will give pitted or lumpy scarring. Temporary darkening around the hair root can occur. Electrolysis on the health service is only available for the face. Removal of all excess hair will require years of treatment and a great deal of expense. It is worth the investment if you are very distressed by your appearance. Hormone treatment will only change the hair for the length of time of the treatment.

Summary

Most hair problems will get better on their own and there is little that the doctor can do to help unless there is disease of the scalp.

5. Imperfections and How to Deal With Them

Scars

Skin damage by cutting, burning or severe inflammation always scars. Surface injuries often heal with temporary discolouration only. Your type of skin determines whether you make inconspicuous scars or lumpy scars (keloids).

The face heals quickly and scars are often unnoticeable. Plastic surgery, if done carefully along the expression lines, makes invisible scars. The backs of the hands heal well, the arms less well, and the legs slowly with bad scarring.

The chest and upper back may produce unpleasant scars which take weeks to heal, and the scars gape and widen. Keloids are common here. Minor blemishes or birth marks should never be removed from these areas for cosmetic reasons as the scar will be worse than the blemish.

Kinds of Scars

Discolouration

Discolouration of the skin is often mistaken for scarring.

Initially, all scars are red, pink or purple. This colour fades over the next year. The blood vessels in a scarred area may be very noticeable.

All colour changes can be camouflaged with make-up or special covering creams.

Keloids and Lumpy Scars

Many scars become temporarily lumpy during healing and later flatten.

Some people form permanently lumpy scars called keloids. These are most common on black skin, particularly on the chest and back. They may form as a result of spots, cuts, earpiercing, but sometimes just appear. If you form keloids you should not have any cosmetic operations as the result may be much worse than the condition you were treating.

Treatment of keloids is very difficult and lengthy. Cutting them out causes a new and bigger keloid. A combination of steroid injections into the keloid with steroid tape and continuous pressure is the most successful treatment. X-ray treatments can sometimes help. Very large keloids are cut out and then immediately treated with steroids or X-rays.

These treatments can *only* be done by a doctor. They are not always successful.

Pits

Chickenpox, acne, boils and insect bites can all leave pitted scars. In acne, both tiny 'icepick' scars and large pits may occur.

Recently, collagen injections have been used for pits and wrinkles. The results can be very good but are shortlived. They may last as little as six weeks, and rarely more than a year. They can cause an allergic reaction, making you ill for weeks.

Dermabrasion can be used for pitted scars and deep wrinkles. A high speed metal brush is used to rub away the skin, down to the bottom of the pit or wrinkle. Dermabrasion of the face requires a general anaesthetic and the skin must be frozen and stiff. It is very damaging to the skin. Afterwards, the face is raw and bleeding, and complete healing takes several weeks. There may be discolouration and sensitivity to sunlight for months. Sometimes the dermabraded area does not blend in with the rest of the skin. The results are usually cosmetically disappointing as there may be flatness and uniformity of the skin, with less skin movement, and altered colour.

Dermabrasion must be done by an expert recommended by your GP or a medical specialist.

Lumps and Bumps

Moles (Pigmented naevi)

Moles are extremely common and harmless lumps in the skin. They are not visible at birth but appear during childhood and early adult life. It is normal to have moles. There may be hundreds of them. Moles vary in size and colour—from dark brown patches to fleshy bumps. In the early stages moles may be inflamed and red, but they eventually settle down and become less obvious. If new moles develop over the age of 35 they should be checked by a doctor. They may become darker and more noticeable during pregnancy, and with the contraceptive pill.

When should they be removed? Very few moles become cancerous. Warning signs are:

An increase in blackness of the mole, especially if the colour is uneven.

Increase in the size of a mole.

Changes in the edge of the mole—an uneven or red edge; tiny black dots around the mole.

Bleeding or ulcers on the surface.

Any new mole appearing after the age of 35.

Itchy moles.

If these occur, see your doctor at once.

Most moles are removed for cosmetic reasons.

Birth Marks

Port Wine Stains. These flat red marks are usually found on the face and scalp. They cannot be removed by cutting them out but laser treatment and infra-red treatment are now being used. They can be camouflaged.

Strawberry Marks. These alarm parents because they develop soon after the baby is born and grow rapidly from a bluish small mark to a bluish-red fleshy lump of blood vessels. They can bleed. The mark increases in size with or faster than the baby but eventually it shrinks. By the age of ten, a white scar will be all that remains. These birth marks must be left alone — however disfiguring and upsetting. Any surgical treatment will cause a worse scar *in the end* than nature.

Stork's Bill Mark. Some babies have a red birthmark on the nape of the neck, known as a stork's bill mark. The hair will cover this.

Dark Patches. Very large areas of brown hairy thickening ('Becker's naevi') may develop on arms and trunk in the teens.

These are impossible to remove, as large scars are left and the naevi return after a short time. Small warty brown birth marks may be cut out but often come back.

Mongolian Spots. Babies of Oriental or Asian origin may have bluish birth marks over the lower back. They are harmless and fade after 18-24 months.

Lumps and Bumps in Adults

Skin Tags

Small tags of skin are very common on the neck and in the armpits and groins. They can be removed by tying a fine thread around the stalk so they drop off. They can be snipped off with sterile scissors or burnt off. Removing them doesn't prevent more arriving.

Seborrhoeic Warts

By the age of 60 we may have lots of greasy warts on the face, neck and trunk. They are brown or black. Frequently people worry about them being skin cancers. They may become itchy and sore, but they are only a cosmetic nuisance. They can be removed by scraping (curettage) or freezing. If there are too many this is impossible.

Skin Cancers

In this country most skin cancers develop in the very elderly. In fair-skinned people the main cause is too much sun. Past X-ray treatment or exposure to toxic chemicals (for example arsenic) are rare causes.

Types of Skin Cancers

Rodent Ulcers. The commonest skin cancer is the rodent ulcer—a pearly bead which slowly increases in size to give a small ulcer. These are usually on the face and sun-exposed sites (see Chapter 1). They do not spread elsewhere but grow until removed.

Keratoses. In old age, these numerous scaly patches appear on the scalp, face, ears and backs of the hands.

Other Skin Cancers. Fleshy rapidly-growing lumps or bumps in the skin may spread to other parts of the body so should be dealt with immediately.

Treatment of Skin Cancer

Skin cancer rarely spreads to the rest of the body but needs to be removed by a hospital specialist by:

Radiotherapy
Surgery, or
Cryotherapy—liquid nitrogen can be used to kill cancer cells by freezing.

The earlier a skin cancer is diagnosed, the easier it is to treat. If you think you have a skin cancer get it checked by your doctor—*don't* delay to see if it will go away, because it won't.

Colour Changes in the Skin

Getting Darker

The skin may darken because of pigments in the skin. The two main pigments deposited in the skin are iron and melanin. Blood is broken down to give iron so bruises may leave brown marks on the body in sites where the circulation is poor—especially on the lower legs and inner forearms. However, the body usually mops up bruises quite well and most forms of brown marks on the skin are due to the deposition of melanin—the naturally-occurring skin pigment (see Chapter 1).

Darkening of the Skin after Skin Disease

Many skin diseases, especially eczema, provoke the colour cells (melanocytes) of the skin to overproduce pigment which drops down into the dermis of the skin and leaves a brown mark when the skin trouble disappears. Even a mild rash may give marked darkening. This is called post-inflammatory hyperpigmentation. Fortunately the body can slowly remove this pigment and most darkening fades over 1-2 years. The darkening is worst in black skin and may occur even after acne.

Once this type of colour change has developed there is little that can remove it except time—best to use a covering make-up and let nature deal with the problem. However, prevention of skin inflammation by early treatment of skin disease will help prevent the colour change.

Melasma

Increased hormone levels in the body during pregnancy stimulate the colour cells of the face and brown patches appear especially around the eyes, on the cheeks and on the upper lip. The contraceptive pill can cause similar brown patches. Naturally-occurring hormones cause the problem commonly in women, especially those of Mediterranean origin, who are not on the pill or pregnant, or rarely in men. The brown patches last for many months but usually slowly fade. It is most important to avoid sunshine which will darken the existing patches so use a total sunblocking cream (e.g. Spectraban forte, Piz Buin 12, Coppertone No 15, ROC 10) over the brown patches, together with a sunshade or sunhat. It is also important to exclude an allergy to perfume if this is a possibility.

Perfume Allergy

Allergies to perfume may produce dark patches on face and neck. These perfumes may occur in aftershaves, cosmetics and creams in addition to perfume sprays. This is often brought out by sunshine so it is important to wash off all perfumes before sunbathing. Once you have developed the streaky brown marks you should avoid sunshine and wear a sunblocking cream when out of doors until the colour fades. Plant allergies also occasionally give brown streaky marks on the skin.

Birth Marks

Most brown birth marks are moles and fairly small. However, some birth marks are very large and brown and more disfiguring. They are often hairy. The only way to deal with this colour change is to have surgical removal but this may be very difficult if the birth mark is large, spreads over creases of the body or is a bizarre shape.

Skin Lightening Creams

In many societies the possession of a white skin is thought necessary for social advantage and the use of skin lightening creams or bleaching creams is very widespread. They all contain a chemical called hydroquinone (in a concentration of 2%-5%) which interferes with the production of melanin. It does *not* remove melanin which has already been formed. Therefore, these creams cannot lighten the post-inflammatory pigmentation which is the commonest cause of brown patches. They can lighten normal skin, birth marks and freckles and unfortunately can also lighten and mask cancerous moles—so *never* use on any brown mark which is increasing in size. Hydroquinone is very irritating to the skin and may produce inflammation with more darkening of the skin, or blotchy discolouration so stop using skin lightening creams at once if any itching or redness occurs. Another problem with prolonged use of hydroquinone especially in high concentration (5% and over) preparations is damage to the underlying tissue leaving black lumps and cysts so only use 2% hydroquinone creams unless advised by a dermatologist. Monobenzyl ether of hydroquinone may contaminate bleaching creams and can cause permanent colour loss which is more disfiguring than the original problem.

A word of warning! Many bleaching creams stocked in West Indian and Asian grocery stores are labelled as skin care or skin tone creams without mentioning their bleaching property. Check the small print for contents of the cream and do not use hydroquinone unless bleaching is desired.

Some skin lightening creams containing hydroquinone:

Artra Skin Tone Cream (2%)
Boots Fade-Out (2%)
Ambi Skin Cream
Esoterica Facial Cream (2%) and Fortified (5%)
Dorot Skin Care Cream
Venus de Milo Cream
Palmers Skin Success Cream

Other Pigments

Other pigments in the skin may cause darkening of the skin,

often of slate grey appearance rather than brown. Workers with mercury and silver in poor working conditions may get greyish skin on the face and hands.

Drugs may cause changes in skin colour which tend to be all over and so do some diseases—liver disease and glandular disease for example. So if you are going brown all over with dark creases of the hand see your doctor.

Very dark patches may develop in later life in the groins and armpits. They can be a sign of illness so you should get them checked by a doctor.

Getting Lighter

Vitiligo

Vitiligo is caused by antibodies killing the melanocytes of the skin which gives clearly outlined completely white patches of skin. These cause little trouble apart from their appearance but unfortunately they often occur on the visible parts of the body, around the eyes, mouth and hands. They are common in people of Asian and Oriental origin where they are more noticeable than in white skins.

It has become apparent that vitiligo can be caused by occupational exposure to nitrophenols and there may be other chemicals as yet unrecognised with similar effects. If several people in your work place have vitiligo bring it to the attention of your Health and Safety Officer.

Coping with Vitiligo It is difficult to stimulate recolouration of the white patches. In a number of cases the colour grows in from the side as little islands of colour which join up but this becomes less likely as time goes on. Your doctor may give you a cream to help in the early stages but the patches are harmless so camouflage is often the best resort. Vitiligo has no protection against sunshine and will burn on sun exposure. Therefore, always use a sunblock on vitiligo in summer. It is a good idea not to sunbathe anyway as vitiligo looks worse on a sun tan.

Pityriasis Alba

Eczema in black children and adolescents may cause

immobilisation of the colour cells and show up on the skin as white patches, particularly on the face. These white patches are not usually china white but slightly coloured. These will get better after treatment of the eczema.

'Post-Inflammatory Hypopigmentation'

Any inflammation of the skin can cause a loss of colour as well as an increase in colour (see above). This is again common in black skins and will clear up on its own given time.

Pityriasis Versicolor

This superficial fungus infection causes circular and scattered areas of colour loss on the chest and back. This is very common especially in those who live or work in hot and humid climates. Treatment of the infection will be followed by a slow recovery of colour (see Chapter 3).

What to do about white patches

Covering Make-up

There are several thick covering make-ups available in chemist shops. 'Covermark', which is used in hospitals, comes in a large number of colours which can be mixed to provide an exact match with your own skin colour. It is advisable to get professional advice from a trained cosmetician as to the exact mix for complete camouflage. The make-up is very thick but will stay in place all day. It can be used to camouflage flat birthmarks in addition to vitiligo or colour changes generally.

False Tanning Solutions

False tanning solutions contain dyes which stick on the surface of the skin and therefore last much longer than make-up. The colour may be rather artificial but some people with vitiligo are happier to use these solutions.

Very Extensive Vitiligo

In people with very large areas of vitiligo it is the normal skin which appears dark so the appearance may be improved by using a bleaching cream on the normal skin. Always avoid sunbathing with extensive vitiligo as you will burn badly.

Cosmetics and Beauty Treatments

Cosmetics are a pleasure to many people. Their benefits, though genuine, are modest and the claims made for them are very exaggerated. Cosmetics are a luxury, not a necessity. Much effort goes into their formulation to make them pleasant to use.

Some cosmetics care for your skin and others are for adornment. Inexpensive substitutes are available but can be less pleasing to use and do not give a sense of luxury, as many people cannot believe they work as well as expensive cosmetics. We are conditioned to believe that we get more for more money.

The skin surface is as dead as our hair. No application to the surface of the skin can alter the dead cells. The most that can be done is to swell the cells with water, i.e. hydrating or moisturising the skin, and to stick the cells down smoothly with greases or emollients.

Cosmetics claim to perform miracles, to prevent aging and wrinkles, to make your skin younger, smoother, thicker or thinner by the use of many exotic ingredients. These ingredients are hormones, vitamins, herbs, collagen, elastin, proteins, and chemicals of strange formulae. Most are of dubious function and value, and if they were absorbed (as claimed), they could cause serious illness.

The array of products available is bewildering. The diversity and ingenuity of the products reflect the major aim of the cosmetic industry, which is to make profits. The constituents of cleansers, moisturisers, day creams, night creams, hand creams, body lotions and foundation creams are all similar. The differences in price do not reflect the cost of ingredients. In more expensive products, only the perfume, packaging and image may be more costly but the ingredients are the same. The chief constituents are oil-water emulsions, i.e. fine droplets of oil suspended in water or fine droplets of water in an oil. The oil-in-water mixtures are lighter, rub in (as the water evaporates) and will wash off with water. Water-in-oil mixtures are thicker and greasier (cold cream is an example), and do not wash off in water. Cosmetics contain water, oil (from plants such as coconuts and avocados or animal or mineral oils), fats (e.g. lanolin), waxes (e.g. bees' wax), stabilising agents and emulsifiers, fillers, colouring, perfumes, and preservatives to stop the cosmetics turning rancid or growing germs.

Cleansers

Soap, cleansing bars, detergents, scrubs, lotions, gels and creams are some of the many ways to clean the skin. All remove surface dirt, grease and dead cells but none 'cleans out pores'. Pores are grease gland openings. These glands cannot and should not be cleaned out!

Once-daily skin cleansing is sufficient. Mild soap and water with thorough rinsing is satisfactory, but if this is too drying, a cleansing lotion or cold cream can be substituted. Greasy make-up and eye make-up require an oil-based cleanser. Liquid soaps (detergents) do not produce a scum in hard water, but can be very drying. The choice of cleanser depends on your preference. There is no one ideal, perfect method.

New bathing products are constantly appearing. A daily bath in winter often dries out the skin; bubble baths and bath salts further dry the skin. Bathing less often, using bath oils and moisturising after the bath prevents this. Aqueous cream (removed with tissues or water) and the heavier emulsifying ointment (used only with water) are both suitable as mild inexpensive face and body cleansers.

Toners, Astringents and Fresheners

These products are promoted for those who feel that the pores of their skin are too obvious. They cool the skin by evaporation and make it feel tight. They do not close the pores. Those containing alcohol temporarily remove grease, making the face matt and the pores less obvious. This effect is temporary as the skin rapidly replenishes the sebum.

Moisturisers

Moisturisers, hand creams, body lotions etc., all work on the same principle. Skin looks its best when containing the maximum amount of water. Moisturisers do this either by applying a water-holding substance (humectant), e.g. urea or polyethylene glycol, or by using an oil or grease to prevent water evaporating from the skin. The greasy water-in-oil emulsions are more satisfactory than lighter oil-in-water ones. These are best applied to skin with a high water content, after bathing, washing or steaming the face.

Central heating dries out the skin by water loss to the dry air.

The choice of moisturisers depends on personal preference. A single moisturiser is enough for face, eyes, lips, neck, hands and body. Night creams are greasier than day creams. Extra 'nourishing' or 'regenerating' ingredients cannot feed dead cells and most do not influence living cells. Cheap substitutes are urea creams (Calmurid and Aquadrate) for hydration, and E45, Vaseline, liquid paraffin and baby oils to prevent water loss.

Most moisturisers also make the skin feel smoother by lubricating it with oil, and make it look smoother by sticking down the fine scales.

Prevention and Treatment of Wrinkles

There is only one way to prevent wrinkles and retard skin aging—a lifetime indoors from dawn to dusk! Sunlight is responsible for skin aging and can only be avoided by daily use of sunscreens and avoidance of sunbathing from infancy.

The only successful treatment of wrinkles is surgical, deep peeling or chemabrasion. Moisturising the skin makes wrinkles less obvious. Make-up disguises them. Creams and potions with miracle ingredients and complex treatments sell hope but no other benefit—because you want them to work you cannot be an objective judge of their effect.

Adornment

Lipsticks, powders, blushers, foundations, eye cosmetics and nail varnish all modify and enhance our appearance. Cosmetics for adornment consist of fine powders and colours for face powder, eye shadow and blushers, or oil-water emulsions with colouring to make foundation, cream eyeshadow and cream blusher. Metallic powders, mica or fish scales provide glitter, pearlised and frosted effects. Lipsticks are basically waxes and colouring.

Are Cosmetics Safe?

Cosmetic firms are required by law to perform extensive and sometimes cruel animal testing to eliminate harmful compounds. Beauty-without-Cruelty products contain only long established ingredients so animal retesting is not required. Some herbal or so-called organic cosmetics contain natural ingredients exempt from testing, but absence of preservatives means they go bad quickly.

Make-up allergies do occur, despite testing, and are discussed in Chapter 2. The most common allergies are to perfume, preservatives and lanolin. Cosmetics which are specifically advertised as hypoallergenic (Almay, Clinique and ROC) omit perfumes and other common allergens, but still contain preservatives and other potential allergens (which cause less trouble—but don't avoid it altogether).

Beauty Treatments

Most beauty treatments are a luxury and provide only a temporary improvement in appearance. They have no permanent effects.

Facial Saunas

A warm bath or steaming the face over a bowl of hot water is as good as a facial sauna; it hydrates and warms the skin, making it look smooth, pink and glowing.

Face Masks

These pastes dry on the face, making the skin feel tight. They remove debris and mildly peel the skin, making it look smoother. Those you buy and those applied in beauty parlours are very similar.

'Facials'

These consist of steaming masks and moisturising, with many exotic extras. At the end of the facial, the skin is clean, smoother, well hydrated, pink and glowing but these are only temporary effects.

In acne facials, the peeling mask and removal of individual blackheads produce an improvement in appearance lasting for several days. They may be very helpful before some important event.

Massage

This is pleasant and transiently increases blood flow, producing a healthy red face, but has no long-term benefit.

Electrical Treatment and Cold Lasers

There is no evidence that these have any effect other than psychological.

Cellulite

Cellulite is subcutaneous fat and responds to weight loss only as a result of diet or exercise, or both.

Peeling

Light peeling uses compounds which destroy and remove the very outer layers of the skin and is beneficial in acne by reducing blockage of the sebaceous glands. It is advertised for fine wrinkling but the claims are unfounded. This must be done with great care and only by experienced people in a salon that has a reputation to maintain. It is much more damaging than a face mask and should not be done at home.

Deep peeling should be done by a doctor and is potentially dangerous.

Tattoos and Cosmetic Surgery

Tattoos

Tattoos are very popular. Teenage enthusiasm for self-decoration often becomes adult shame and embarrassment.

Removing tattoos is difficult and unsatisfactory as the tattoo is replaced by a more unsightly scar.

Removal must only be done by a doctor, otherwise disasters occur. The tattoo can be removed by:

1. Cutting out the tattoo.
2. Dermabrasion (see scar section), replacing the tattoo with discoloured, hairless, rough skin.
3. Salabrasion—superficial dermabrasion using salt.
4. Laser—a new, experimental treatment which scars. Lasers are dangerous and should only be used in hospitals.
5. Infra-red—very intense heat applied to the skin is quick and simple but leaves scars.

Cosmetic Surgery

Cosmetic surgery and other procedures for removal of birthmarks, moles, scars, and the effects of aging, must be done by your GP or a dermatologist, or a plastic surgeon recommended by them.

Moles

Removal of moles causes scarring and distortion. It is often better to keep your 'beauty spot' than trade it for an unnatural scar. Cutting out is most successful along expression lines on the face, but on the back and chest the scars are worse than the mole. Electrical burning (cautery) of the mole leaves a pit. Surgical shaving, where the mole is cut off flat to the skin but not completely removed, can give initial good results, but is not suitable for hairy moles. The hairs can be removed by electrolysis.

Birth Marks

Flat Port Wine Stains are best expertly camouflaged. Your local hospital will have a clinic for this. Surgical treatment is useless. Laser treatment is promising but should only be done at an NHS hospital as in inexperienced hands it can be an expensive way to buy a nasty scar. The results have been shown in a large series of patients to be cosmetically most acceptable when the patient is adult and has a dark purple stain—too late for most teenagers who are deeply unhappy with their birthmark. A test area is done and the results assessed some months later. The treatment takes many sessions over years. Infra-red treatment which is used at a few centres is giving promising results.

Broken Veins

Electric cautery is treatment used for prominent red veins but may scar. Lasers and infra-red can be used.

Scars

Unsightly scars from accidents or operations can sometimes be improved by a plastic surgeon. If he or she feels unable to help, accept this advice. Do not pay someone to make this scar worse.

Wrinkling and Furrowing

Cosmetic surgery for the effects of age can be successful, but you must know and understand the limitations and risks beforehand, otherwise you will be disappointed.

Consult your GP who will recommend a good plastic surgeon. You do not want an inexperienced or unscrupulous surgeon. Successful cosmetic surgery will make you look younger but will NOT stop you continuing to age.

The most successful and least risky operation is removal of bags under the eyes and drooping eyelids (blepharoplasty). Face lifting is more hazardous, leaves scars and may not obliterate all wrinkles.

Chemabrasion

This is a combination of deep peeling by chemicals and dermabrasion. The skin is chemically destroyed down to the dermis (as in a burn). The face swells up like a tomato and is very painful. New smoother skin forms over the next few weeks.

Deep peeling is potentially dangerous and should only be carried out by a doctor with wide experience and training in this technique. Such experts are rare in the UK. It should NEVER be done by a beautician.

Although it removes wrinkles around the eyes and furrows around the mouth, the results can be disastrous and even fatal if it goes wrong. The new skin may be discoloured, or, at worst, scarred permanently.

The risks, discomfort and a high cost seem too much to pay to look five years younger. The face will continue to age despite the treatment.

All cosmetic procedures have risks. Interfering with the skin chemically, physically or surgically will scar it. For minor blemishes the anguish caused by the scar is worse than the original defect. If you are considering such a procedure, discuss it with your general practitioner, dermatologist or plastic surgeon. Often it is best simply to use covering make-up, or accept yourself as you are. Results of surgery seldom look drastically different to the outside observer, and may look unnatural.